Dr. Dan's Last Word on Babies and Other Humans

Dr. Dan's Last Word on Babies and Other Humans

DANIEL G. HELLER, MD
&
NANCY S. HELLER, MSW, JD

Dear Hilary,
I very much enjoyed talking with you at dinner. Clearly, your interests and Dan's are similar and I am very much looking forward to the Heller lecture tomorrow. I hope you enjoy this book and best of luck on your next publication!
Best,
Nancy

iUniverse, Inc.
New York Lincoln Shanghai

Dr. Dan's Last Word on Babies and Other Humans

iUniverse books may be ordered through booksellers or by contacting:

iUniverse
2021 Pine Lake Road, Suite 100
Lincoln, NE 68512
www.iuniverse.com
1-800-Authors (1-800-288-4677)

The views expressed in this work are solely those of the author and do not necessarily reflect the views of the publisher, and the publisher hereby disclaims any responsibility for them.

ISBN-13: 978-0-595-42038-4 (pbk)
ISBN-13: 978-0-595-67964-5 (cloth)
ISBN-13: 978-0-595-86383-9 (ebk)
ISBN-10: 0-595-42038-9 (pbk)
ISBN-10: 0-595-67964-1 (cloth)
ISBN-10: 0-595-86383-3 (ebk)

Printed in the United States of America

In loving memory of Dan,
who lit up my life
and the lives of so many

Contents

Acknowledgements

Dan and I were writing this book at the time of his death. Together, we had intended to dedicate this book to our deceased parents, Hon. Philip and Mildred Heller, and Drs. Martin and Rose Grundfest Schneider. We were both fortunate to have such loving and supportive parents.

Dan also wanted to thank Dr. John Herrin. Dan greatly admired Dr. Herrin, a pediatric nephrologist who was Dan's mentor, beginning during Dan's residency in pediatrics. John, a first-rate clinician, had taught Dan how to acquire clinical and diagnostic skills and Dan believed that his pediatric training was enormously enhanced by John.

Since Dan's death, our long-time friend, Jim Russek has been the force behind bringing this book to publication. He has encouraged and supported me (and my children) during the difficult days since Dan's death, and he also views this book as his friend's legacy. He has been a bridge between the publishers and me and he is responsible for the title and cover. I have valued his good opinions and advice and am very thankful for all that he has done.

We sought advice and information from many pediatric specialists about several topics in this book. Dr. Mark Pasternack, an infectious disease specialist at the Massachusetts General Hospital for Children, edited the chapters on immunizations and antibiotics. Dr. Allan Ropper, Chief of Neurology at St. Elizabeth's Medical Center in Boston, improved the sections on brain function. Dr. Ronald Kleinman, a pediatric gastroenterologist at the Massachusetts General Hospital for Children, weighed in on nutrition for babies. Dr. Tracey Daley, a pediatrician and colleague of Dan's at Centre Pediatric Associates, reviewed several sections of the book and provided advice and information about growth and development. Dr. Judith Willner provided advice about genetic issues. Dan consulted Drs. Mari-Kim Bunnell and Angeli Kaimal about the chapter on birth. Our niece, Pamela Heller, edited sections and we valued her helpful advice and contribution. I am sure that there are others from whom Dan sought advice; unfortunately, I do not have their names and can only thank them anonymously.

Dr. Sasha Helper and Prof. Alan Hirshfeld played a key role in the initial effort to publish this book and they have provided editing and enthusiasm for this project before Dan's death and since. Tom Curtis also offered constructive editing advice. He and Sandy Sheehy gave generously of their time and counsel about writing a book. And Susan Ellis provided much needed assistance with contract issues.

After his death, Dr. Dan's patients and their parents overwhelmingly responded to my request by writing their stories about Dr. Dan's relationship and advice to them. Those stories have become the heart and soul of this book. The recollections of patients and parents depict Dr. Dan's personality, style, and humor in poignant and vivid language and keep loving memories of him burning in all of us. My heartfelt thanks to them and to all who helped bring this book to publication.

Introduction to Dr. Dan

Dr. Daniel G. Heller was a practicing pediatrician in Brookline, Massachusetts, for twenty-eight years before his sudden death on November 12, 2004. At the time of his death, he and I were writing a book on pediatrics, an advice book with physiological explanations, lessons that Dr. Dan had learned in his own life, and stories about our parenting and what we have learned.

Dan had important and sage advice for today's parents and wanted to share that advice with a wider audience beyond his practice. Why? From his observations during his twenty-eight years of practice, he saw that today's parents are significantly more anxious and less confident about their own child-rearing skills than those young parents whom he first encountered when he began practicing pediatrics.

Today's young parents are often far away from their own families and don't have access to the experience-based advice of elders. With moms and dads working outside the home, young parents have less community support today than their counterparts twenty-eight years ago. Dan viewed today's medical system as encouraging less dependence on parental common sense and more dependence on the providers of medical care and advice, such as lactation consultants, pediatricians, and pediatric specialists.

For instance, he wanted parents to understand why the current push to breast-feed babies soon after birth is wrongheaded and why new mothers shouldn't be discouraged when they can't breast-feed immediately. He wanted parents to understand that all babies are prone to gastroesophogeal reflux and that this normal physiological occurrence doesn't have to be treated with medicines and surgeries. He wanted parents to relax and enjoy the upbringing of their children and to understand that most stages of childhood are within the realm of normal.

But why should today's parents read yet another book filled with pediatric advice? After his death, hundreds of letters, cards, and e-mails poured in; those communications from parents of his many patients documented Dr. Dan's care and concern for his patients, his diagnostic acumen and wisdom, and his unique and humorous style of relating to both parents and children—his laugh-out-loud style that made his patients want to go to their doctor. Those stories provide you with some idea of the unique human qualities Dr. Dan Heller possessed in abundance and of the message he wanted to communicate to a wider audience. He called himself Crazy Dr. Heller, and this book is his legacy—filled with very sane advice that can make a difference in your parenting.

Crazy Dr. Heller

Parent Cristina O. wrote,

In February of 1998, my son was twenty-three months old and was scheduled for surgery to receive a Cochlear Implant (a device which assists deaf people to hear by converting sound waves into electrical impulses that can be recognized as sound). I was in the parent waiting room area after Christopher's surgery began. All of a sudden, I hear this squishing sound coming from down the hall. Squish, squish, squish and who appears around the corner? A gentleman wearing nylon snow pants and a bicycle helmet with a propeller on it.

"Hey there, Cris," (as he called me). "It's just me, Crazy Dr. Heller. What time will Christopher be done?"

I didn't know he was coming in and I was so flattered and surprised that he had. He hung around for a quick minute and then had to go about his day. I told him that he is nuts to ride his bike in this weather; he agreed and we laughed. He said, "I'll be back later on."

And sure enough, while Christopher was in the recovery room that evening, again we hear that squishing sound and there is Dr. Dan wearing the same outfit, helmet and all. I recall the nurse looking at me and I said, "It's okay; that's my son's pediatrician."

"Hey there," he said, "I am just here checking on my little guy; I want to know how he did."

He brought my son Christopher something we cherish and hold dear and will always remind of us this memory and all the other memories and stories we have. It was a Propeller Beanie just like his. There in the hospital bed is my son with his head all bandaged and wearing a propeller beanie. Did we laugh!

We will never forget "Crazy Dr. Heller." He always went above and beyond.

Meeting Dr. Dan for the First Time

Parent Beverly L. wrote,

My first encounter with Dr. Heller was at an Open House (a newborn information sessions for expectant parents). Of course, I had no idea who Dr. Heller was and when I saw this funny grown man sitting in the waiting room (at Centre Pediatrics) with a colored striped hat with helicopter blades on top, I for sure thought, "Is this where I want to be?"

I loved Dr. Heller's speech about Centre Pediatrics and its philosophy. His honesty and candor weaved along with his training, intellect, and experience intrigued me so. I chose Dr. Heller based on his whimsical, charismatic charm. In reality, I think it was his hat that did it. I think I was mesmerized by it and fell into a trance.

Parent Christine H. wrote,

Dr. Heller was our oldest son's pediatrician when we lived in Boston.

We moved to Florida in 2000. I just heard about Dr. Heller's death and am very saddened by it. He was a wonderful pediatrician. Although we only knew him for the first two years of Michael's life, Dr. Heller left a lasting impression on us. Much of the advice he gave us we still remember vividly today.

We visited an open house at Centre Pediatrics when I was still pregnant. Dr. Heller was there that night. He asked the parents if they had any questions. One woman asked what the best density was for a child's mattress. Dr. Heller responded (approximately)," Let me see, most children are born in the rice fields on the ground. What is the density of the earth? I guess that is the best density." After that answer, my husband, Hannes, and I knew Dr. Heller was the perfect pediatrician for us. His no nonsense attitude, let's not overcomplicate the matter and throw our brains and logic out the window just because we are going to have a child, appealed to us.

Parent Jamie L. wrote,

I first met Dr. Heller when I was a nurse at Children's Hospital. I was standing at the desk, retrieving lab results from the computer when this man with a "beanie cap" and a "Rotor Rooter" shirt with the name "Dan" on it walked behind the desk. Needless to say I was surprised and asked him if I could help him. He then proceeded to inform me that he was a pediatrician here to visit one of his patients newly diagnosed with cancer. Two things struck me at that moment ... What a cool guy and I want him to be my kids' pediatrician. I proceeded to tell every person I came in contact with that day of my experience. The next day I called and switched my children's care to his practice. He was not accepting new patients at the time but I figured that anyone who was "ok" with Dr. Heller was "ok" for us.

Parent Kim S. wrote,

I had my first, Aiden, in December 1999. Dr. Heller was the pediatrician doing rounds that day and he appeared in my doorway wearing: a propeller rainbow hat, shorts, t-shirt, totally full backpack (it was HUGE), a whistle and sneakers. He may have had more, but it was enough that I thought he was a singing telegram!

He said something along the lines of "Hi, I'm the pediatrician on rounds today. Let's take a look at your baby..."

To which I replied laughing, "Yeah, right, let's see your identification!"

Obviously, he was who he said he was and I was eating a very large piece of humble pie as he examined Aiden and accepted us as new patients.

It makes me smile EVERY time I think about him and thought maybe it would make someone else laugh too. He had the child-at-heart personality that shined through.

Parent Dean I. wrote,

Our firstborn bundle of joy arriving into this world with two "horns" on top of his head. During the birth process, the doctor had to attach two suction cups to his head and yank him out.

A week later, it was discovered that his mother, my wife, had a severe bleeding problem which required a return to Brigham and Women's Hospital for diagnosis.

So there we found ourselves: Mom with this scary thing that even the best doctors were having trouble figuring out, seven day old Luke, with two horns sticking from his head, and Dad, helpless and seriously concerned about the whole situation, sharing a small hospital room.

It was anything but the typical joyous entry into parenthood.

On the second morning, while Mom and Luke still slept, I heard a knocking at the door. When I opened it, the room's darkness was brought to light by the glow of the man in the shorts, high-top sneakers, ankle weights and beanie hat with the propeller. Needless to say, we all know who that describes.

In his Dennis Miller like delivery Dr. Daniel Heller introduced himself. "I'm here to see young Skywalker."

I wheeled the crib to the door so as not to disturb my sleeping wife.

With grave concern, I pulled back the sheet from the sleeping Luke.

"Dr. Heller," I said, "I'm really concerned by his head. I ... I ... I'm concerned about these protrusions."

Dr. Heller reached down to each one and acted like he was squeezing them while making a nasally honking horn sound.

"You know Dad, he looks like the statue of Moses outside the Vatican, the one where he has the horns ... That's pretty impressive."

Of course the image was dead on, and for the first time in three days, I broke a smile. Then returning to business I asked "Will they go away?" "Well, if they don't you can always buy him a hat." And he smirked.

"Don't worry Dad, young Skywalker is going to be just fine. The horns will go away. You have a perfectly healthy child. Take care of Mother and you guys will be out of here soon probably without the horns ... The statue of Moses ... That's pretty good."

He smiled, shook my hand and walked away. "I'll check back with you in a day or two." To this day, looking back on that tense time, I still have to smile at how his humor broke the incredible tension that our young family was feeling.

Parents Robert and Patricia L. wrote,

We met Dr. Heller the morning our newborn son, Charlie, and I were being discharged from Brigham and Women's Hospital. By the luck of the draw, we learned that a fellow named Dan Heller had done the pediatric exam, and he came by the room. He was wearing a beanie with a propeller, a Chicago Bulls T-shirt and extremely short cargo shorts. Perhaps because it was a summer Sunday, and perhaps because of the doctor's attire, my husband assumed that the doctor was a resident "who just happened to go to medical school a little late in life." Dr. Heller told us that Charlie's *bilirubin* was a little high, so he wanted us to stop by Centre Pediatrics the next day. When we got there my husband learned that this fellow in the propeller hat, bulls T shirt and short shorts was not a resident, he was the guy in charge! We soon also learned that he was the best pediatrician a child could have.

Parent Linda Y. wrote,

Tom, Mike and I loved Dr. Dan. I wish we had told him. I know we thanked him after each visit but not in the way we wished we thanked him. We didn't say, "You are our favorite doctor. You made a difference in our lives. You are smart and wonderful and we love you."

Visits with Dr. Dan became EVENTS that we always looked forward to, enjoyed, and learned from. The first visit was always a shocker. Dr. Dan undressed our infant gently, held him one-handed above his head, then ran around the waiting room at Centre Street yelling, "Flying naked baby! Flying naked baby!"

The commotion that erupted was a sight to see … toddlers screaming, parents in hysterics and us—the owners of the kid—in disbelief. This was the very first lesson in not taking ourselves too seriously as parents.

Dr. Bruce Bunnell told this story at a memorial service for Dr. Heller:

Several years ago, while I was rounding at one of the Brigham and Women's Hospital nurseries, a new father shared a funny story with me.

Early the previous morning, this new father went to the hospital lobby in search of coffee and bagels. While waiting in line at the coffee shop, the father noticed a man enter the lobby. He was struck by the odd appearance of this man. In the midst of a brutally cold New England winter, this man was dressed in a bicycle racing shirt, shorts, ski socks pulled up to his knobby knees, ankle weights, a hospital ID badge around his neck, and a propeller attached to the top of his bicycle helmet.

Just the sight of this character made such an impression upon the new father that, when he returned to his wife's hospital room, he told her about his experience. This new dad worked in the human services field and was very impressed that the hospital was so progressive as to hire such an obviously mentally challenged person.

About ten minutes passed when the new parents heard a loud knock on the hospital room door. To their surprise, shock, astonishment and horror, the same man walked into the room, complete with the propeller helmet, shorts, ski socks, ankle weights. Now the man had a stethoscope around his neck and was pushing a portable crib with their new baby!

Greeting the shocked and befuddled new parents, the man proudly announced his arrival. "Hi, I'm Dr. Heller. I'm your pediatrician and am here to examine your baby."

Dr. Dan was, without a doubt, the most unique, charismatic and outgoing individual who one will ever meet. As one mother remarked to me, "You will always remember the first time you met Dr. Dan."

Dr. Dan's Diagnostic Skills

Susan K. L. wrote,

Dr. Dan was an original—that's the only way I know how to put it. And, we are heartbroken that he is gone. He is such a huge part of our family history that memories keep flooding in. For example, when Elizabeth finally slept through the night after months of disturbing our sleep, Julian and I were not only shocked: as new parents, we were also *worried*, if you can believe that, that her brand new sleep pattern might signal a serious medical problem. Dr. Dan was on when I called, and I will never forget how he questioned me closely about symptoms and listened very carefully to all I said. Then, as I hung on to every word of diagnosis he could provide for me, he slowly explained, "That, Mrs. L., is what we in the medical profession refer to as ... a blessing!"

As soon as I had digested the reality that Elizabeth was okay, I felt such relief and had a good laugh, too. This was our introduction to Dan's genius. By way of humor, he helped us to save face and realize at the same time that we shouldn't take the normal ups and downs of life too seriously. Voltaire once wrote, "God is a comedian playing to an audience too afraid to laugh." I think Dr. Dan understood that, and he could laugh, and he could make us laugh, too.

But always, always, you could count on his medical judgment, and that was key. For example, we brought Elizabeth to Dr. Dan with a complaint about a sharp pain in her side. Tests showed no particular problem. After Dan had pronounced her healthy and was ready to send her home, he noted that she stood, bent over, with a pained grimace, against the wall of this office, her hand gingerly holding her side. He said, "That's not right," and without further ado, sent us to a surgeon for an appendectomy. After the surgery, the pathology report showed appendicitis. You couldn't let the humor fool you: Dan was a doctor who listened closely to his patients, who read the body language, and who acted quickly when speed was necessary.

Interestingly, Elizabeth's appendicitis also formed the backdrop for one of Dan's political assaults on the medical system. He had a hard time connecting with the surgeon of his choice because of insurance red tape. He later showed me a letter he had written blasting a system that would prevent this young girl from getting the medical attention she needed. I will never forget his outrage at the system and his proactive stance to do what he could to fix it.

Our middle son, Jeff, is currently in medical school. As a patient, Jeff was the beneficiary of Dan's teaching, when Dan would pull a medical text off the shelf to help explain the reasons why Jeff had a sore leg, a sore throat, or any other complaint. There are not many pediatricians who would take the time to nurture a kid's interest or respond to them.

When our youngest, Jonathan, needed a shot for a summer trip to Brazil, Dan encouraged Jonathan to open his eyes to what he might be able to see, learn and do in Brazil. What a great lesson from a man who, with all of his knowledge about disease, might have emphasized constricting caution over openness to new adventure.

Writing about Dan in this letter helps to keep him close to us, and ending the letter feels as if we have to let him go. But the truth is that we will never really let Dan go from our hearts or our memory. The L. family, like so many others, have been indelibly affected by Dan's tremendous expertise, his incomparable sense of humor, his contagious love of life, his enormous heart, and his persistent concern for justice in the medical profession and elsewhere. Simply put, Dr. Dan Heller was a giant.

Parent Jennifer G. wrote,

When our daughter was born at term, she was sent to the NICU and diagnosed with severe laryngomalacia (a life-threatening condition in which tissue of the larynx collapses into the airway). After a week of tears, stress and several meetings with ENT and NICU staff we were scared and exhausted.

Dr. Heller was the only one who looked at us squarely and with a wave of the hand said, "Don't worry, leave her alone—she'll be fine," which gave us the confidence to bring her home and take over as her parents. And he was right. She is now an energetic (read: unstoppable) two year old who has never had any breathing-related difficulties.

We will never forget the confidence and compassion that Dr. Heller provided us.

Parent Sharon A. wrote,

Our memories of Dr. Dan are so sweet and so full of happiness. After my son's pre-college visit, I had planned to write to Dr. Dan thanking him for taking such good care of our children. Of course, I didn't get around to it, thinking I had plenty of time. Now I can only hope that Dr. Dan knew how much we valued his common sense, quick intelligence, and sense of humor.

When Hardy would have his checkups, Dan would goof around. He would engage Hardy in some sort of joke, extra large needles or whatever to trick me when I came into the examining room. There was always lots of laughter.

On a more serious note, he correctly diagnosed our daughter, Lura, fifteen months at the time, with bacterial meningitis. Her illness had been labeled as an ear infection by another physician. We remember that Dan sat Lura on the floor where she promptly fell over.

He said "Kids, this ain't no ear infection. Go to the hospital. I am calling ahead to tell them to expect you for a spinal tap."

He saved her life. There were not and are not enough words in any language to thank him sufficiently.

Dr. Dan's Relationship with Children

Parent Sara B. wrote,

For Andrew's six-month-old checkup, I had dressed him in a plaid lumberjack shirt. When Dr. Heller saw Andrew, he said: "That's the kind of shirt a guy likes to wear!" I really don't know why that struck me and stayed with me all these years, except that perhaps it is just one little example of how fun and engaged and lively Dr. Heller always was.

Most people say they'd rather do a lot of things than go to the doctor, but my son and I always looked forward to our visits with Dr. Heller and were sad when they were over. For several years during Andrew's checkups, when Dr. Heller would ask Andrew what he wanted to be when he grew up, Andrew would say "marine biochemist." After a while, Andrew must have wanted to catch Dr. Heller off guard, because when asked about his future profession, he would try to think of ever wackier career choices (e.g., bartender) just so that he could amuse Dr. Heller and have a lively conversation with him. We loved his sense of humor, and always wanted to amuse him too, when we could.

When my daughter Sylvia came along in 2001, she grew to love Dr. Heller too and always wanted to stop and say hi to him even when her appointment was not with him. On one such occasion, we were waiting in the lobby for Dr. Heller to wander by so that we could say hello. Sylvia, about two years old, was in the habit of wearing a gold plastic crown on her head upside down—points pointing downward. Dr. Heller came walking by. He stopped, said hello and remarked at what a WONDERFUL idea it was to wear the crown upside down and that everyone should try it. He said that he was going to wear his hat upside down too. He took his propeller beanie off, flipped it over, put it on his head upside down, and walked off. You can imagine how delighted we both were.

We were very fond of Dr. Heller, and we are selfishly sad that we can no longer see him and enjoy his wonderful style and brilliant way of practicing medicine. Having Dr. Heller for a doctor was like having Mary Poppins for a nanny. How wonderful he was at taking care of our kids and putting them at ease. Cliché as it may be to say, he really was one of a kind.

Parent Jody L. wrote,

My first memories of Dr. Heller were when I was just a young girl and my mom would take me and my brother to Dr. Cohen for our annual physicals.

There was this very young, hyper man, running around Dr. Cohen's once quiet office, and I remember whispering to my mom" Is that really a doctor, mom?"

When, my kids were born, Sam in 1988 and Kate, in 1990, it was a given that I would use Dr. Cohen as my pediatrician. And I remember bringing Sam in for his first visit at two weeks old and seeing that young, hyper doctor running around a busy pediatric office and thinking ah, yes I remember.

Well the years passed and Dr. Cohen retired, and we naturally started to see Dr. Heller. Because Dr. Cohen threatened my son with an extra shot if he didn't behave himself, my young kids were a little nervous to meet this new doctor with the colorful beanie on his head. Needless to say, both kids loved Dr. Heller.

When Kate was small, Dr Heller asked her if she wanted to have a boy doctor or a girl doctor. She said girl, and so he examined her wearing a hat that had a long braid attached!

Parent Beth B. wrote,

Going in for regular checkups was always something the kids and I looked forward to—unlikely for me because my hands even sweat when I take the dog to the vet. At each visit, Dr. Dan would have one zany hat or another perched on his head—braids, beanie copter, fireman hat, etc. and be going about his business with a sense of purpose and a twinkle in his eye. Just waiting to see if Dr. Dan was wearing the bike helmet with eyeballs (if he had just come from the hospital) or conversing intelligently as Kermit the Frog was enough to take the sting out of needles and fear out of doctor's visits.

Parent Elizabeth W. wrote,

Alex is seventeen and has been a patient of Dr. Heller's since he was six years old. No matter how sick Alex may ever have been, when we visited Dr. Heller, Alex always left feeling better. Dr. Heller just had that way with kids.

The last year and a half had been very difficult for Alex ... During his visit to Dr. Heller in August, Dr. Heller shard his own experience with his first heart attack and his thoughts on stress, coping with difficult situations and being on therapy. He encouraged Alex to continue in therapy and to try to develop a positive outlook on life.

I remember when we arrived for that appointment and had to sit in the waiting room for our turn. There were several loud, screaming young children. Alex was a bit annoyed and I made the comment, "Well, now that you're seventeen, this will be your last visit here; we'll have to find you an adult doctor."

Alex replied, "Dr. Heller's not an adult?" We both laughed at this thought.

Patient Doug F. wrote,

In the past 17 years that I have known Dr. Heller, I can't recall a time when I asked a question of him that wasn't quickly, but nonetheless thoughtfully, responded to with some joke about my developing body, soul, or mind. Maybe the response wasn't even funny; maybe it was just his propeller hat that always put a smile on my face ... who knows. Sadly enough, I have another question that I would like to ask my pediatrician today, but he's no longer here to deal with my queries. If he was though, I would ask him, "Dr. Heller, how come there are so many evils and wrongs in this world, but still such sadness is cast upon the beautiful, brilliant, giving, and caring?" I can picture him answering too, "Well Douglas, why don't you find the tallest ladder you can find, climb up, ask God, then climb back down and get back to me because I'm dying to know myself. For now, let's talk about your beautiful sisters."

Patient Tarek K. wrote,

As a child I was never very fond of trips to the doctor's office. I always associated them with bad news, and, more pressingly for a rather rotund ten year old, admonitions against things I liked (cola and donuts) and prescriptions for things I didn't (running laps). When I saw Dr. Heller, it was different. Full of cheer, charm, and humor, he had a way of making visits to the doctor's fun. Not just fun, in fact, but funny.

Dr. Heller was blessed with a wit and a sense of humor that could bring a smile to any upset child's face. He was completely disarming, and within minutes of stepping into the examining room, you were too busy laughing and talking with him to notice that he had taken your blood pressure and given you a tetanus booster.

I recall once when I was eleven coming in for a checkup, and somberly explaining a school project to raise money for victims of Chernobyl. "Isn't that a tuna factory?" he exclaimed. By the time I had convinced him that Chernobyl was in fact a nuclear power plant, the visit was over and I was out the door. Trips to the doctor's office were painless when Dr. Heller was in.

Most importantly, however, was Dr. Heller's presence and humor when he was on call. When it is late at night and something happens, one is always struck by an alarming sense of panic. This was when Dr. Heller was always at his best, when his ability to put everything into perspective and to make one feel calm was most important.

One evening, while I was babysitting my brothers, I received a nasty crack to my nose in a tussle. I was convinced that it was broken, and, moreover, that this was a crisis. I called Centre Pediatrics, and Dr. Heller called back. As I explained what had happened through the layers of tissue that swathed my bleeding nose, he asked one key but pointed question: "Are the boogers shooting out in strange directions?" When I had ascertained that no, the boogers were not coming out in strange directions, he assured me that my nose was fine, and to forget it. I went to bed that night very pleased that I had handled the situation "maturely" and quite happy that the Dr.'s advice had included the word "booger."

Dr. Heller was a brilliant pediatrician who knew so well how to relate to his patients, and furthermore their parents. He mixed humor and professionalism, good advice and wit, and most of all, made you feel that everything was going to be okay.

Patient Gabriel R. wrote,

I have known Dr. Heller since my memory began: there are few people outside my family that I can say that of. His advice, concern and guidance over the years changed the way I grew up, and the way I have lived my life. He taught me when to be serious, but also the power of levity. He coaxed out an inner confidence: helping me take care of myself as well as my health. He helped me understand the importance my actions had on myself and others.

Dr. Dan taught me at a young age to while away time by placing random calls to 1-800 numbers. They were toll free, so what was the harm? Come up with a good seven letter phrase, dial it, and see who answers. He put his phone on speaker and dialed and tried 1-800-DEARGOD from his office. The telephone rang and rang and then a recorded message came on, "the number you have called is outside of your calling area." Dr. Dan had a ready answer, "No kidding. You have to be clergy."

He was a wonderful man, and I owe him an incredible debt of gratitude.

Patient Nicole G. wrote,

I am now 26 years old, so it has been a long time since I have visited Dr. Heller's office, but I still have such great memories of him.

I would always make a fuss and gag when it was time for Dr. Heller to stick that big wooden stick on my tongue to look down my throat … he would go crazy yelling "bad stick" "bad stick" and he'd break about 20 of them just to get me to laugh. He always had a way to make the bad things fun! He could have easily doubled as a comedian!

Patient Christa M. wrote,

Dr. Heller took the time to get to know all of his patients. Before every appointment he would sit me down in his office and ask his favorite line of questions: What was my favorite color? What was my favorite food? What did I want to be when I grew up? And, of course, every year he had to make several jokes before the appointment was over. I remember one year he taught me how to answer the phone when I was home alone. He began by asking me how I currently answered the phone when no one was home. I said, "Well … I don't know." So he began his simulation of the situation:

Dr. Heller: Ring. Ring. Ring. *Ring.* Well come on now Christa, you have to pick up the phone!
Me: Um, hello?
Dr. Heller: Hello, is your mom or dad there please?
Me: No. Can I take a message?

At this point, Dr. Heller made a funny face at me and I started laughing. He said, "No, no, no. Whenever someone calls for your parents, never say they *aren't* home, say something like 'Sorry, my mom's in the shower right now' or 'Sorry, she's in the bathroom with explosive diarrhea. Can she call you back?' That one *always* works.

Dr. Heller was constantly joking around. I remember once when I had to have my finger pricked; I was really nervous. Dr. Heller sensed my anxiety and he put a piece of scotch tape over his ear. I looked at him like he was crazy and he said, "Look Christa, I'm listening to a tape. Get it? Scotch tape, tape?" Of course I started laughing and felt more relaxed.

Dr. Heller was an exceptional pediatrician, friend, and mentor. We will always remember the beanie hat he wore on his head, the weights he wore on his ankles, but most of all we will remember the love he had for his job and his patients.

Patient Nicholas M. wrote,

I went to Dr. Heller's office for my yearly physical and he sat me down in his office before the appointment; he said he had a great trick for me to try. He began by telling me that he was on vacation and it was his birthday. Everywhere he went he told people that he was 50 years old today. He said it was funny because he didn't tell anyone that it was his birthday, he just told them how old he was on that day and magically, everyone assumed it was his birthday. He told me that he got a free dessert and a free drink! Every time that I'm in a restaurant and hear that it's someone's birthday, I smile; I think of Dr. Heller.

Parent Jackie W. wrote,

My sons have felt the same about Dr. Heller from babies through eighteen years old. They thought Dr. Heller was always "cool" through all those years. There are not too many people that teenagers meet that never lose their coolness but Dr Heller was one of them … He gave my sons 120% at every visit and phone call but more importantly, he really cared.

Parent Joni S. wrote,

Dr. Dan's charisma was unique; I had never seen a doctor wear a whirly bird hat before. But his magnetism became clear when our daughter was almost

2. One day, while eating raisins, she proudly announced that she had put one up her nose. I was unable to retrieve it so we came to the office and Dan got it out. He made lots of jokes, had Jenny in hysterical giggles, and ended the visit with a hug which Jenny eagerly returned.

The next day, Jenny put another raisin in her nose. I asked her why she would do that again and she told me that she wanted to see Dr. Heller "right now." So back to the office and more hugs and giggles. On the third day, I retrieved the raisin myself.

As Jenny got older their relationship maintained a special closeness, so much so that Dr. Dan promised Jenny that she could see him until she turned 21 or graduated from college, whichever came first. It was a promise that, despite insurance hassles, he kept.

Recently, Jenny told me that she had called him several times while at college because of a minor heart problem Dr. Dan had discovered when she was 18. She told me that he always took her calls. I was not the least bit surprised.

With every shot came a kiss, an explanation, an apology for the pain; I truly think he felt a pinch with every vaccination. With every visit, came reassurance and love for the children he treated and respect for parents' efforts to raise their children. No question was ever stupid, no concern disregarded.

Through the years, we have had our share of issues like every other parent but some, like the time David (our third child) had an anaphylactic reaction to an antibiotic on an airplane, were particularly harrowing. We landed in Florida and took an ambulance to the hospital where five strange doctors worked on our four year old. I called the office and within seconds Dr. Dan was on the phone to the doctors in that Florida emergency room. He continued to talk with them throughout the days that we were in the hospital. The Florida doctors were flabbergasted; they had never had so much contact with an out of state doctor regarding a kid's care. I told them how special my pediatrician was. They told me that I was more than lucky.

Parent Debby B. wrote,

My son, Jeffrey, aged 8 or 9, and I came to the office for a sick visit. The receptionist told us that it would be at least 40 minutes before Dr. Heller could see Jeffrey. She asked if we would like to see another doctor.

I knew that my son would be impatient. "Why don't we see someone else," I suggested to Jeffrey, who was never good at waiting for anything. "Dr. Heller is busy."

Jeffrey frowned and looked at me like I was crazy. "We'll wait," he said, matter of factly.

Nothing would deter him. He was going to sit in that reception area until Dr. Heller was ready to see him. And I wasn't going to argue with him. If he was my doctor, I thought to myself, I'd wait forever to see him.

Parent Georgette N. wrote,

I never let my 17 year old son know how I felt but it was funny to see him sitting in the waiting area surrounded by infants and toddlers. Dr. Heller never discontinued his hat-change routine with Burgess, who at first, always seemed slightly offended that he was being treated like a "child" but always ended up laughing his way through the appointment. The hat changing would continue even during our serious discussions about Burgess going into the Navy.

Parent Dotty B. wrote,

We always loved the developmental questions Dr. Dan asked the kids in his office before each annual exam and learned quite a bit from their answers. At various stages of their development, the kids focused on Dr. Heller's funny hats, the bike he rode to work, and the wonderfully irreverent comments he made, thereby taking the seriousness of the visit completely away. They actually enjoyed their checkups and never dreaded sick visits.

Dr. Dan's Relationship with Parents

Parent Suzanne M. wrote,

We often discussed things not directly related to modern medicine and these discussions will have the most lasting effect on our family. There were many times that we would ponder the greater meaning of life and Dr. Heller would dedicate more time to those conversations than to the routine physical exam. One particular story will always stay with our family. On one occasion I shared my concern about my son who was having difficulty reading in his earlier years. I was very worried that school would always be a challenge and wondered how that might affect his pursuits in life. Dr. Heller took out a blank piece of paper and wrote the initials MMR on it. [Editor's note: In this context, MMR stands for mildly mentally retarded.] Dr. Heller then shared a personal story about how teachers labeled him (as MMR) early on in life. He went on to explain that he drew enormous strength from that misdiagnosed assessment of his skills. He shared this story as an example of how a child's support system can change his outcome in life. I will remember that conversation always and there were many days that I drew strength from it.

Parent Dr. Andree H. wrote,

I was fortunate enough to meet Dan during my residency at Massachusetts General Hospital. During my emergency room rotations, I always looked forward to, and enjoyed, the evenings during which Dan, as attending physician, would be our teacher. I enjoyed and learned to appreciate his common sense approach to practicing pediatrics.

He was also extremely honest and humble. I remember one evening when Dr. Heller called a patient's mother, within earshot of several of us residents. He apologized to this mother because he felt he had missed a finding on her child's exam and in retrospect, he felt a different course of action should be taken. That event stands out as one of the few times (and possibly the only time) I saw any attending physician appear willing to admit (to a patient, in front of residents) that he may have been wrong about something.

I was so impressed by Dr. Heller that I chose him as my children's pediatrician. This is a choice I never regretted, even when it meant traveling one and one-half hours each way to his office for appointments. Despite the fact that many thought of him as a brilliant comedian of sorts, Dan wasn't afraid to let a sensitive, caring side, show through. And despite acknowledging the fact that I too am a pediatrician, he allowed me to just be a mom when it came to my children.

Dr. Heller would always make an effort to make children and parents feel very comfortable and cared for. As Robbie and Nicole approached their teen years, I can remember him telling them, "You know you have your parents, but you have Dr. Heller too … and you can always pick up the phone and call me if you ever have a question."

Parent Jen B. wrote,

As a new mother, I remember the first time Dr. Heller came to check on my son in the hospital just after he was born. He came into the room and I was thinking to myself, "Why is that bike courier picking up my baby?"

Since then, I always expected the unexpected when it came to Dr. Heller and I looked forward to each visit with my three boys. Even my sister, who had never met Dr. Heller, would always look forward to my stories after one of my sons went to see Dr. Heller. In addition to his unique sense of humor, Dr. Heller always made me feel like I should use and trust my instincts as a mother. Rather than preach how to care for my children, he often asked how I thought I should do things and then usually told me to do just that—within reason of course.

I believe he genuinely respected the role of mothers.

Parent Lynette S. wrote,

Dr. Dan had a wonderful way of calming an hysterical mother. When Daryn fell out of her high chair, I was completely and utterly hysterical. I rushed her into the office and Dr. Dan examined her. He then told me that she was absolutely fine, "although she might not go to Harvard," he quipped. We laughed and I left the office feeling a huge sense of relief.

When Alex developed a high fever, I was hysterical and over-wrought again, and called the office to make an appointment with Dr. Dan. He had just come back to town and was still on vacation, but he came into the office to see us! (I still marvel at that.)

He examined Alex, and reassured me that my son had a virus, and would be fine, "although he might not go to Harvard either," Dr. Dan joked. Again, we shared a good laugh. Dr. Dan had a unique and humorous way of reassuring a high-strung parent!

Parent Christine H. wrote,

Dr. Heller was an amazing pediatrician, but he was more than just a doctor. He seemed to me to be a philosopher who happened to also be a wonderful pediatrician. He understood our society and what information/advice parents needed to raise their children. I remember him saying that parenting is not rocket science and that women have been doing it for thousands of years.

Our children will tell us when they need something. We don't need to read books to know what children need; we just need to listen to our children.

Parent Stacey L. wrote,

My husband and I attended an open house during the last months of my first pregnancy. Dr. Heller made a statement that has stuck with me ever since. He said, "For every parenting book that tells you to do something one way, you will find just as many that tell you to do the opposite. As parents, you should not find this confusing, but instead find it liberating." I cannot tell you how many times that has been replayed in my head or how many times I have shared it with friends and family.

Parent Melissa W. L. wrote,

I cannot tell you how much my family and I miss Dr. Dan. Every time the annual visit comes up, or we have a questionable night with our now 8 year old daughter—we always ask ourselves, "What would Dr. Dan do?"...... My husband, Joe, always says, "If Dr. Wappa Dappa was hear, I'd bet he'd say....", and it would be something to make us laugh and take a deep breath, and know that everything would be okay. I don't know how Joe came up with that name. He has a habit of naming people, and having an internal code, a code that only he and Jaida understand. Dr. Wappa Dappa became their term of endearment for Dr. Dan, and it just stuck with all of us.

You know, I always think back to when I was about to deliver our daughter. I remember not taking the time to find a pediatrician before the birth. Jaida came 2.5 weeks early, and I was panicked about not having completed this important task. I prayed to God that the person who saw her in the hospital would be kind, compassionate, love kids, and have a great personality, and have lots of experience. Well, the day she came, and a man walked in with a weird helicopter hat on and shorts.... I just watched him. By the time he finished talking with Jaida, and talking with me, I KNEW he was the one. My husband kept saying, "'HIM?' are you sure?"...... I was so absolutely, positively sure. Joe always joked about the many hats our dear Dr. Dan had. I loved to play with them during our office visits. And so did Jaida. As much as Joe joked about those hats, he knew that Dr. Wappa Dappa meant business.

From the time when Jaida swoll up like an 'oompa loompa', to us torturing her with 3 shots and an ear piercing at 4 months; and still to her later years of toddler fascination with her newfound 'female parts' and announcing it throughout Disneyland (and everywhere else), Dr. Wappa Dappa always had a story to share which would make me laugh and know that she would be okay.

I worried about what she would eat at under 1 year of age, after weaning her. He let me know that if she were in China, perhaps she would eat rice and fish, so don't panic; if she were in Italy she would have pasta; and if she were in Africa, perhaps she would have potatoes. He let me feel okay bringing a two page list of questions to each session … and he answered them.

By far, my favorite memory however is that as Jaida got older, still as a toddler though, she would address him as Dr. WappaDappa … and he responded to her as such. I remember when she first began questioning her body, and Dr. WappaDappa shared his story with me of his own children parading around the house giving a "P&V" show! I felt okay that my kid seemed to be preoccupied with confirming that every woman and girl had the same parts as she did.

I appreciated the time he took with her, and with me, helping me feel confident in raising a bright little girl.

Dr. Dan's Advocacy on Behalf of Children

Parent Joan W. wrote,

Dr. Dan joined our battle with an uncomprehending insurance company which denied our daughter access to the only medication which worked in fighting a severe dust mite allergy while failing to offer a sensible alternative. This battle was frustrating and time consuming for us and Dr. Dan, and included Dr. Dan's instructing the hapless insurance clerk in more medicine than he ever wished to learn, and resulted in our receiving permission to have this particular medication as necessary through the year 2999!

Parent Victoria K. wrote,

My son has seizures. Last year, my son's school principal was trying to take away summer school and bus service from him, but Dr. Heller told me and the school principal that *any* child can have a seizure, not just my son. He also said the school (if the nurse is not available) and the bus driver should call 911, if my son has a seizure at school or on the bus. The principal did allow my son to go to the summer school on the bus because of Dr. Dan.

Practicing Pediatrics in Dr. Dan's Own Style

Parent Victoria K. wrote,

Dr. Heller respected and care about my family and my culture. He learned and spoke some Chinese like 'Good boy', 'Good Girl', 'Hi', and 'How are you?' He always returned phone calls. I can always feel his love for my children as if they are his children.

Parent Kelley T. wrote,

I have had a special place in my heart for Dr. Heller ever since my oldest daughter was 9 months old. Rather than send us to the hospital after office hours one night, he had us bring Julia to your home so he could tend to her nursemaid's elbow. He sat her on your kitchen counter, took care of the problem, and proceeded to have your dog Woody perform for us.

I have told that story over the years many times and people are just amazed: above and beyond the call of duty.

Parent John S. wrote,

We first met Dan many years ago at our first visit to him with Julie, age 3. During the stethoscope exam, he decided that he needed the assistance of his nurse, and called for her in a pretty fair Jack Benny imitation. He then reached in his desk and pulled out a nurse puppet, to which he talked for a while, and then attached to the scope. This performance put Julie at great ease, but afterwards made me ask my wife Barbara whether she had checked to see if Dan had actually gone to medical school. Finally, the Ladies' Home Journal named him as one of the best pediatricians in the USA in 2002, and I stopped worrying.

Dan told us a story: When he and Alan Dershowitz, a Harvard Law Professor, attended the same hospital reception, Dershowitz spotted Dr. Dan, with his propeller hat and shorts, from across the room. Dershowitz walked up to Dan, and said, "You know, my experience is that a man who chooses to look so strange in such august company is either a lunatic or exceptionally gifted."

Parent Judith S. wrote,

I looked forward to my kids' appointments with Dr. Dan the way someone looks forward to a planned right of entertainment—I'm sure I'm not alone in that feeling. Dr. Heller had a way of cutting through the bullshit, getting at core truths, global and timeless truths, suddenly realigning everything into the bold starkness of a new perspective. He was blunt without being disrespectful. And everything he said came with the authority of his years of practice and ample book knowledge. Mostly, the emotional effect of talking with him was one of relief that everything would be okay, and it always was. We wish we could thank him for injecting life and humor, wisdom and knowledge, integrity and kindness into our children's first encounters with medicine. Dr. Dan Heller was a lovely man.

Friend Jen B.-L. wrote,

One of the first things Dan said to me after Alex was diagnosed with autism was that he didn't like labels and that all children are unique bundles of strengths and challenges. Our job as parents is to help them use the former to overcome the latter. One of the second things he told me—and I can see him standing before me in your kitchen, we were cleaning up after another one of your wonderful meals and he looked at me with warm, sad eyes and gave me a hug and said "Boy, I wouldn't want to be in your shoes."

To me those two statements taken together—and combined with the example of how Dan lived his own life—have been key to coping. The second statement was a frank, honest and warm-hearted admission that we were living something that was incredibly painful and difficult. Because he acknowledged the validity of my pain, I could accept his first statement as something more than simple platitude. I didn't want to be in my shoes either but I was and Dan had given me a high-level road map for coping. Don't bog down in labels and diagnosis and prognosis—move forward, right away, one step at time. Savoring and building on Alex's strengths to tackle the rest.

Parent Barbara L. wrote,

In 1988, my son, Alex, was born with a unilateral cleft lip and palate. Although it was only seventeen years ago, and although it occurs in one out of seven hundred births, neither my obstetrician or pediatrician, Dr. Heller, had experienced this birth defect with any of their patients. Everyone was at a loss for words.

In the first twenty-fours hours after having my son, I was in a complete daze. Little could be done to console me. The shock of having a child with a facial deformity was one that I was unprepared for. Obviously, so was everyone else at Beth Israel Hospital. No one knew what to say as they scurried around trying to figure out how to feed this new little baby who couldn't nurse nor use a conventional bottle. My door was kept closed, with only caregivers allowed in. Dr. Heller showed up the next morning, checked Alex out, assured me he seemed otherwise healthy. He did a lot of listening. Even he was speechless!

Nurse after nurse came in to sit with me and tried to think of something to say that would temporarily relieve my pain. One said, "Well, at least he has all of his fingers and toes." Another followed with, "You're lucky he has both arms and legs!" One night nurse even told me that I should feel fortunate that my son wasn't born mentally retarded. These comments felt artificial, and certainly didn't relieve anything. I did not want to feel "lucky", knowing that other children had been born with worse. This felt bad enough to me and I wanted someone to understand that. Even a family member, upon entering the room and seeing Alex for the first time exclaimed, "His head is so round!" as if that would make me feel better. It angered me that no one could be honest with me about how hard it was to look at this child and to imagine what he would have to go through at such an early age. I just wanted to be left alone.

The next morning, Dr. Heller showed up, as he did every morning thereafter. On this morning, he sat on the couch in my room. I will never forget that moment. He said to me soberly, "I don't know what to say to you. I have talked to my colleagues to try and get advice about what to say and how to handle this. All I can say is that you have a kid who is hard to look at; but he won't always be that way. Surgery will do wonders to help him regain some of what was lost to him. It will get better, but for now, it will seem very, very hard."

I just cried. "Finally, someone is honest with me" is all I could think of. I felt relieved. I wasn't crazy. I wasn't so fragile that people needed to dance around the obvious. Dr. Heller was never known for sugar coating his message … and how I loved him for that. At that moment, I knew we were stuck with each other. I would never have my son see any other pediatrician, and I knew I could consider Dr. Dan as our partner in helping Alex develop and overcome whatever obstacles might face him.

Well, my hopes, and prophecy, came true. Throughout the first year, and two surgeries later, Dr. Heller checked in with us at those most important times. After eight weeks, and Alex's first critical surgery, Dr. Heller **BIKED** over to our house **after** work so that he could see that Alex was okay. House visits? … unheard of!

Over the years, and as Alex grew up, he loved his visits to his doctor. He would always be guaranteed a laugh with the beanie-wearing "crazy" Dr. Heller. And Alex learned, too, to be honest when Dr. Heller would ask him all of those questions: Can you count? Do you read books? Can you kick a ball? And the most important: "What does your daddy do?" Alex enthusiastically answered, "He climbs big mountains!" Dr. Heller would follow with, "What does your mom do?" Alex proudly said, "She shops!" Well, upon leaving that appointment, Alex received his first of many mommy lectures on ALL of the things that mothers do besides shopping!

It is hard to think of a world without Dr. Heller. Alex will forever think of Dr. Heller, the personality larger than life, with a smile on his face. His beautiful, amazing, effervescent face! Dr. Dan was with us from the beginning and he will be in our memories until the end. And, in the L. family, Dr. Dan's spirit, his childish enthusiasm, and his love of children, and his passion for honesty will follow his memory for years to come.

1

Pediatricians: A Simple Definition

During the interviews for a new pediatrician for our practice, I ask each applicant, "What is a pediatrician?" After four years of medical school and at least three years of residency, all candidates answer that a pediatrician is a doctor who takes care of the medical issues that arise between birth and adulthood. When I finished my formal training many years ago, I am positive that I echoed that same idea.

Now, after eight years of academic training and over twenty-five years of practice, I realize that the job description is much more complex. As any given day begins, I am not sure, as a pediatrician, exactly what I will be or what I am.

Hospital Rounds

I arrive at a hospital early in the morning to see newborn patients on the maternity floors. Today, I will examine ten newborns, and each one will have a unique story. I enter the room of a one-day-old infant and find his new mother in tears because her nursing is "not going well." A breast pump is attached to her breasts, and her baby is contentedly sleeping in a bassinet. I wonder why she has a breast pump. Why in the world is she nursing a machine instead of relaxing after the stress of childbirth? On exam, this newborn is beautiful and normal; yet the mother is crying because she feels like a failure. I spend twenty minutes being a lactation consultant (see chapter on breast-feeding).

In the next room is a teenager who is giving up her baby for adoption. The teenage mother seems calm and resolved; her own mother is in tears. The grandmother-to-be is distressed and depressed beyond words over losing her grandchild. I spend thirty minutes being a social worker and a psychiatrist.

1

In the third room is a baby with a funny-looking face and other odd features, which raise the possibility of Down's syndrome. The findings are not definite, and only a chromosomal study will provide the definitive answer. I have to inform the mother about this potential lifelong problem and also tell her that we won't have an answer for several days. What should she tell her relatives and friends? How would she feel? I spend another thirty minutes as a geneticist, psychiatrist, rabbi, and friend for someone I have never met before.

In the fourth room is a mother whom I know; she has two other children who are my patients. She hugs me and is delighted to have a third child. After I examine the baby and assure the mother that her baby girl is normal, she has no questions, and I am on my way in a few minutes. The next six visits are equally varied.

Back to the Office

I arrive at the office almost on time. A note on my desk tells me to call a mother. Her son fell and went to the emergency room because he has a piece of glass in his thigh. An x-ray shows the glass fragment, but the radiologist in the ER also raises a question of a tumor in his bone. My mind races to think who we can call to review the x-ray. I wonder how the ER physician could send this boy home without an answer for his mother since the ugly issue of a tumor has been raised. I wrote some e-mails and made some phone calls to find out quickly whether another radiologist agrees with the tumor theory. Three days later, the hospital finds another radiologist who reads the film as benign developmental abnormality of the bone.

During the day, patients with urgent problems are given same-day appointments with me or speak with me on the phone. These patients include a depressed mother of a six-week-old, a tearful mother with a teenage daughter who calls her derogatory names, a boy who received twenty-two stitches in his face after walking through a plate-glass sliding door because he was totally spaced-out on marijuana, a divorced father who does not want to pay his bill since he thinks his ex-wife purposely pretends that their two-year-old is sick, and a child with possible attention deficit disorder, whose parents wish to discuss the treatment alternatives. I talk with a young man who just wants my help choosing a college and another who is afraid of dying but who came in complaining of fatigue. At every "sick" visit, my role changes to that of Sherlock Holmes as I try to piece together oral and physical evidence in the pursuit of a diagnosis.

At "well" visits, parents bring issues that must be discussed. Parents have concerns about constipation, language delays, motor skills, terrible twos, toilet training, and eating issues. Each of these visits required me to change my "hat" and become what was needed to deal with the problem at hand.

The Accurate Job Description

"What, then, is a pediatrician?" By the time I ride my bicycle home, I have figured out the answer. A pediatrician is not only a doctor, but also a cardiologist, a neurologist, an endocrinologist, a behaviorist, a social worker, a lactation consultant, a psychiatrist, a dietician, a nutritionist, a father or mother figure, a teacher, a rabbi, a priest, a mentor, and so on.

While most physicians treat patients with a particular problem, pediatricians take on a newborn and provide care and counsel for nineteen years or more. While most physicians have one individual as a patient in an exam room, a pediatrician's exam room is overflowing with a patient and several family members. While most physicians take on diseases and illnesses, pediatricians also take on health and wellness. While most physicians can talk to their patients, pediatricians have to wait for two and half years before their patients can talk. While most physicians take care of people for only one phase of their lives, pediatricians take care of individuals when they were newborns, toddlers, preschoolers, adolescents, and young adults. We are jacks-of-all-trades and have no boundaries on what we need to know. Indeed, what makes my day so great is the fact that I don't know what will come my way. I am challenged from the start to the finish. As Yoda might say, "Boring my life is not."

"Houston, we have a problem!"

Modern medical economics has put a great deal of stress and pressure on a pediatrician's time and on his ability to use technologies and therapies. Despite the multiple issues and patient needs to be addressed, the amount of physician time has been divided between patient and administrative functions to a much greater degree than even fifteen years ago. Economic factors have become a major driving force behind the type and level of medical care that you will receive. Reimbursement is focused on specific guidelines, pharmacy protocols, and documentation of care in a patient's medical record rather than the traditional level of contact between patient and doctor.

What are the outcomes when we focus on cost savings and administrative guidelines rather than on individual patient needs? Here are a few examples:

- We pressure mothers to make milk in two days when that is impossible. In 1974, a new mother was allowed to rest and recover. On the second day, a hospital aide brought Marissa in and told Nancy to begin nursing if she wanted to for about two minutes on a side. Now we tell new moms to begin nursing immediately for longer periods mostly so we can discharge them in forty-eight hours. This saves the insurer money, but the rush to nurse is not physiologically possible. It causes moms to have very sore nipples and, most distressingly, leaves mothers feeling like failures.

- Primary care physicians are encouraged to diagnose attention deficit disorder in their offices. Years ago, insurance companies covered this type of evaluation in learning disability clinics. These clinics were fully staffed by neurologists, psychologists, and education specialists who administered psychological tests and collated teacher and parent information as part of a complete evaluation. Now, many insurers won't cover these "education evaluations." Significant numbers of families cannot afford them, so these complex assessments have fallen into the offices of pediatricians who have inadequate time and resources to complete a thorough evaluation.

- We prescribe medicines not based on efficacy, but on economic efficiency. Many payers now determine which antihistamines and antibiotics are "preferred" by establishing formularies which detail which medicines are favored and which are not. If I prescribe non-formulary antihistamines or antibiotics, an insurance company may question my prescription, and my office may lose economically on some managed care budgets.

- We allow intermediaries to decide what psychiatric support an individual needs. In the past, I was able to make a direct psychiatric referral. A parent and I would discuss the problem, and I would then match a good therapist for a particular situation. Now psychiatric referrals are done by insurance companies. A few years ago, the mother of a ten-year-old male patient threw the father out of their home when she discovered that he was having several affairs with both male and female lovers. My patient tried to throw himself in front of a moving car on the Massachusetts Turnpike, and his mother called me for advice. Obviously, this suicidal boy needed some immediate psychiatric help. The family's insurance company only approved one group therapy session scheduled for ten days later. Sadly, the only psychiatric intervention offered for a suicidal boy was a delayed group therapy session.

- More recently, we are being asked to fly by the seat of our pants when we could fly by the seat of current technology. Unlike thirty years ago, sophisticated tests are now available to assist us in diagnosing cancers and other serious conditions. But providers are pressured by economic factors to avoid "expensive" studies. Currently, at least one insurance company in the Boston area requires physicians to telephone an administrative company to obtain permission to order magnetic resonance imaging (MRI) studies. The mere fact that a physician who orders clinical studies needs prior authorization from a person who has not even seen the patient is intimidating. In addition to the questions raised about their clinical judgments, physicians also object to the additional administrative burdens, which lessen the amount of time spent on direct patient care.

Time is of the Essence

The Beatles said, "Love is the one thing that money can't buy," but they equally well might have said, "Time is the one thing that money can't buy."

The general trend in health care is to spend more provider time on administrative functions than we did when I began practice. We are focused on documentation, risk management, and cost savings in prescribing and testing. Those functions take time. Obviously, the time has come for direct interaction with patients. And the health-care system rewards those physicians who are good documenters and cost savers rather than good "docs" and "mentors."

When I trained at New York University Medical Center, one of the attending (supervising) physicians was Dr. Franz Vogel, who was seventy-one years old. He had been the personal physician for Baron von Rothschild and Sigmund Freud. During one teaching session with four other students and me, he spent more than three hours interviewing a patient and performing his physical examination. During our subsequent discussions, he told us the man had cancer of the gall bladder.

"Could you not feel the odd texture of the gall bladder?" he asked.

Numerous tests on this patient did not establish a diagnosis. Five days later, at an exploratory laparotomy, the patient's cancerous gall bladder was removed. I will be forever in awe of this physician who made a complex diagnosis just by a history and a physical. Clearly, a key ingredient of being able to make the correct diagnosis was time. Dr. Vogel took substantial time in gathering a history from the patient and in examining him.

Technology Saves Time

We have come a long way from the three-hour history and physical to the almost instantaneous information available through our technology. On the simple diagnostic level, for instance, we can now test for strep throat and have an answer in several minutes; years ago, we had no answer for three days.

During my residency in pediatrics, I saw the introduction of the CT scan. When I first began at Massachusetts General Hospital, if a child came in to the emergency room with head trauma, a pediatrician examined him, and then a neurologist was called to see the patient. A history and physical exam was completed, and decisions were made about whether to admit and observe the patient or send the patient home.

Toward the end of my residency, a patient came to the emergency room with head trauma; and before the neurologist or neurosurgeon even examined the child, a CT scan was performed. By the time the specialist saw the patient, he already knew whether or not there was a fracture or brain tissue damage. The diagnosis was made quickly and efficiently by a machine, and the doctor could either admit or send the patient home with confidence in the diagnosis. Today, CT scans and MRIs have significantly advanced early diagnosis and treatment.

A Pill for Every Season and Reason

In addition to the advances in technology, the number of pharmacological agents has increased dramatically. Today, more parents seek the medication solution; they have been led to believe that if no medicine is prescribed, then the condition, symptoms, or illness has not been treated. Doctors prescribe, and patients seek medications for many conditions. Antibiotics are prescribed for viral illnesses despite the fact that antibiotics are only effective in fighting bacterial infections and medications or over-the-counter preparations are available to treat every burp, belch, and fart. If sneezing, a child may be classified as allergic, and antihistamines are recommended; if vomiting, a baby may have gastroesophogeal reflux and is prescribed antacids; and if fussy or crying, a young baby may have colic, for which antacids are also prescribed. For every symptom, we have a pharmacological treatment, whether by prescription or over-the-counter. In too many instances, prescribing a medication is quicker than having a conversation.

The Fast Life

We live in a fast-paced world, and our expectations are fast paced. Physicians live in the same world. Antibiotics are prescribed for a child with otitis media or sinusitis. Frequently, those antibiotics are unnecessary because most otitis resolves without medication, and sinuses do not exist in children younger than six years of age. Parents need and should have full explanations to understand and accept these concepts. However, full explanations require time, and the quicker road is to treat. Unfortunately, this approach has led to more and more antibiotic-resistant bacteria.

For a baby who is spitting up, I spend twenty to thirty minutes explaining to parents that reflux is normal in infants less than ten months of age; I usually illustrate by drawing a diagram of an infant's esophagus and stomach. For a fussy baby, I spend a similar amount of time explaining that colic is a normal and predictable developmental stage (see Chapter 11 and Chapter 13). When parents don't understand the normalcy of these infant behaviors, the sad consequence is that, forever, they believe that their children have some medical abnormality.

We are on the fast lane from the moment of birth when new moms are encouraged to nurse their babies in the very first minutes and hours after the baby is born. Our rush to push mothers to make breast milk in the first few days after childbirth has had the disappointing effect of decreasing rather than increasing the number of moms with successful nursing. The goal has been to foster nursing, but the result has been to stymie it (see Chapter 5).

Technology has clearly shortened the time to get answers, and pharmacology encourages a "quick fix," but humans still need time to understand explanations of symptoms that are within the boundaries of normal and to consider treatment options when their symptoms exceed those boundaries. We, all too often, want to rush the conversation aspect of medicine since "talk" time is not as well rewarded. In modern medicine, actions speak louder than words.

Time Flies by When You Are Having a Good Time

Again, the pace today is a far cry from the three-hour evaluation by Dr. Vogel. Many doctors see more patients per hour than ever before. Current technology gives us fast answers, and modern pharmacology gives us fast treatments. Both patients and providers are on the fast lane to diagnose, treat, and cure.

Unfortunately, most of the problems of infancy and childhood do not lend themselves well to this fast approach. In medical school, I was taught that each developmental milestone and every illness has its own natural history. Chickenpox is infectious for seven to ten days, croup is worse at night and continues for four days, most babies need thirteen months to learn how to walk, and breast milk "comes in" between four and seven days after childbirth. Despite our technologies, these natural histories remain as true today as they were thirty years ago. Some bodily processes just take time.

Time to Slow Down and Talk

We must take a more measured approach to the technological and pharmacological fast lane and return to a more sensible and slow approach for many childhood developmental and illness issues.

This book is intended to empower you to avoid the quick answers. Specifically, I hope to debunk some of the pseudo-diagnoses and treatments that our current health-care system has spawned.

This chapter began with my definition of what a pediatrician is supposed to be. Many pediatricians today are unable to meet this job description because our physician training programs do not teach students and residents how to answer the questions that new parents will pose. Furthermore, in addition to the fact that they are only taught the quick answers, pediatricians feel forced to push off these duties onto lactation consultants, nutritionists, and specialists as a way to save time and keep up with the expected patient volume.

"Houston, can we solve our problem?"

For years, my colleagues and I have expressed our concerns about these factors but basically have done little to remedy the situation. Our job description leaves little time for us to find the "time" to try to change the world. I decided to write this book to try to help you and your pediatrician save some "time." The information is simple and practical. It is the same information and approach I try to teach medical students and young house officers. If you spend the time to learn about nursing, colic, toileting issues, feeding issues, fever in children, and a myriad of other topics discussed in this book, the "time" you spend with your pediatrician will be more directed and satisfying for both of you. The time-saving quick answers will not be necessary. We won't have to invent cures for non-diseases, and we can feel more confident in our child-rearing abilities. We can discard labels like colic, lactose intolerance, and sleep disorders, to name a few, and get back to enjoying our children instead of categorizing their supposed defects.

- A pediatrician is a resource with many talents. Take advantage.

- Many quick answers are not suited to childhood problems.

- Time is not on the side of the parent or pediatrician. Both must make the time.

- By definition, normal is more common than abnormal. Normal infants and children behave in normal ways; treating symptoms that are normal is the wrong way to address the health needs of children.

2

Birth: A Most Unnatural Act Today

Rarely, in the United States today, do women deliver by natural childbirth. We have gone about as far as we can go to distance ourselves from "natural" anything.

Even without a science background or a book, we can imagine what a natural birth must have been like over the past ten thousand years. How did our cave woman ancestors deliver a baby? A quick look backward will empower women to go forward with confidence in their ability to manage childbirth and nursing. In fact, such a backward glance will strengthen an understanding that for the first three days after birth, newborns have little need to nurse, and as with our cave woman mother, little should be expected of today's new mother other than to recover from the delivery of her baby.

The Great Human Drama—There Ain't Nothing New Under the Sun

Birth Drama Act One: *Surprise!*

To begin the story, our cave woman does not know she is pregnant, and she does not get multiple prenatal visits and advice. She knows something is happening because her body habitus is changing over time, and she is just not herself. Her abdominal girth is increasing, and she feels more tired and hungry than normal. She sleeps fitfully and feels uncomfortable in certain positions. Finally, after thirty-seven to forty-one weeks, she starts to feel ill. She has intermittent cramp pains and loses her appetite for food or water. Her pains become longer and stronger over time. What she does not know is that for the next twelve to twenty-four hours, her symptoms will worsen. She is in labor and "labor" it is. She's working hard, and yet she is not eating or drinking. She is becoming dehydrated, and her blood sugar levels are under stress. At times, her pain will lead to moments of panic or unconsciousness. When the pains are awful, she grits her teeth and clenches her hands to distract herself.

Birth Drama Act Two: What a Unique Way to Introduce a New Actor on the Stage!

Finally, the blessed moment arrives. A newborn infant is pushed and shoved out of the uterine world and into our world. Is this the end of the story? No. Our mother, dehydrated and hypoglycemic, now has to separate her circulation from that of the infant. The cord has to be cut; and most likely, our cave woman did not bring a surgical knife or scissor to the event. She has to bite through the umbilical cord that attaches the placenta to the baby just as other mammals do. She then ties off the cord to prevent the infant from bleeding.

Birth Drama Act Three: Oh, Please, Not Again!

Unfortunately, the worst is yet to come. Fifteen to twenty minutes after the delivery of her baby, cramps and pain return, and the placenta begins to separate. Like her newborn, the placenta needs to be delivered; from our cave woman's point of view, the delivery of the placenta is like starting the process anew. The placenta is finally pushed out, and now a more threatening and possibly fatal crisis ensues. The highly vascular surface of the uterine wall, to which the placenta was attached, is similar to an open wound that is bleeding profusely. To the insults of dehydration and hypoglycemia, we add a life-threatening hemorrhage. By our modern definitions, we have a patient who is going into shock; and unlike today, emergency services did not exist ten thousand years ago.

Will a superhero come to the rescue and save our cave mom and cave baby? Luckily, that superhero exists and is known then and now as good old Mother Nature.

Birth Drama Act Four: The Most Unusual Dinner Scene Ever

The very placenta which nourished the cave infant for nine months is now the source for the oxytocin that will induce uterine contractions and stop the bleeding. Our cave mother now eats the placenta and receives nourishment as well as pharmacologic compounds that curtail her hemorrhage.

I will always remember when our Siamese cat gave birth to quintuplets in our apartment in New York City. One by one, she licked her kittens and chewed through their umbilical cords. When all were breathing, she ate the placenta, and her bleeding ceased. Most mammal mothers use their placentas as their source for oxytocin.

At this point in the birth process, an acute hemorrhage may have been controlled; but our cave mother is *still* dehydrated, exhausted, and weakened. She will need a few days to recover. In her condition, she may not be of very much help to her newborn baby. Indeed, to add insult to injury, the situation is further complicated by the fact that our new mother had no milk and, furthermore, will not make milk for three days.

Birth Drama Act Five: The Crisis

NEW MOTHER (*looking tired and worried*): Where is my milk?

MOTHER NATURE: There is no milk; a little colostrum maybe, but definitely no milk.

"What? She has no milk?" If this were a play, the director would instruct the actors to stage this as a tense moment. But this is not a play. The new baby has arrived, and we have nothing to feed it. This is reality, and the truth is that the very hormones that sustained our cave woman's pregnancy actually block her ability to make milk. She will have no milk for three to four days. Our new mother will need to drink plenty of fluids over the next few days to wash out these lactation-blocking hormones. Until these hormones are removed from her body by urination, all she has is a small amount of colostrum. The colostrum is rich in antibodies but does not provide much liquid or nutrient volume. Yikes, is all lost again?

Birth Drama Act Six: Mother Nature Saves the Day

"No breast milk for the baby on day one, two, and three!" Once again, our super-hero, Mother Nature, has a solution. Fortunately, infants are born with extra fluid on board to sustain them for three to four days while their mothers recover. The source of this extra fluid is the fluid in the babies' lungs. While in the uterus, a baby "breathes" in and out; but instead of air, he "breathes" in amniotic fluid. Upon delivery, he takes his first breaths; and in doing so, the amniotic fluid in the lungs is forced across the pulmonary capillary bed and into his circulation. Not only is that fluid enough to sustain the baby for several days, but it also provides the mother with some time before she is really needed to take over the nourishment of her infant. In fact, despite the enormity of the task of delivering a baby, our cave woman has succeeded with a truly "natural" childbirth. While birth is a difficult undertaking, Mother Nature provides aid and support at the proper moments.

Critics Loved Birth Drama in Six Acts

Mammalian reproduction has been very successful, an incredible feat not just for humans but for all mammals over the eons of life on earth. Childbirth has its life-and-death moments, and yet a solution for many of its crises is provided at the moment that the solutions are needed. This system has worked most of the time; that fact is obvious since our species has survived. Childbirth is as real for mothers today as it was for our cave woman ancestors. The lead role is that of the mother, and the supporting role is that of the newborn. All mothers are fully equipped to handle all the details that her role demands even though most have had no specific training to act this part. Women have successfully delivered babies in an unscripted fashion for thousands of years. Childbirth is the longest running drama on planet Earth, and pregnant mothers are going to play the lead role successfully.

Improvements: Birth Drama in Modern Dress

One of the great achievements of modern medicine has been the development of obstetrics as a specialty. Obstetricians have been able to close the gaps in our reproductive system—gaps which can lead to maternal or fetal death.

Today, mothers and fathers learn about the birthing process in classes. Most mothers in the developed world deliver in a hospital or birthing center and are given intravenous catheters to provide fluids adequate to prevent dehydration. That same fluid contains sugar to support the efforts of the "labor" that will end with the birth of a newborn. Pain-relieving medications are available to lessen the pain of the cramps. People are present, including the father, to provide emotional support to the mother. Obstetricians and midwives tie the umbilical cords to save mothers from biting through them. Rather than have the new mother eat the placenta, we inject oxytocin to stimulate the uterus to contract. Our hospitals provide a more comfortable and supportive environment. Our new mother probably feels much better at the point of delivery than her cave woman counterpart.

Most births on this planet occur the good old-fashioned, "natural" way in many parts of the world, including the third world and developing nations. In such countries, as well as in industrialized ones, where hospital support is more common, we have not and cannot change the physiology of our modern-day mother or the physiology of our modern newborn baby. The delivering mother and the newborn infant are no different than the original players in our drama. Just as ten thousand years ago, today's mothers need time to clear lactation-blocking hormones, and today's newborns need time to urinate off the excess fluid in their bodies before they feel hunger and a need for fluid.

Insuring Against a Flop: Doctors, Hospitals, and a Supporting Cast of Thousands

I do not argue that "natural" is better or has fewer complications for the mother and the infant. That is by no means true. Mothers and/or their babies died at a significantly higher rate before the assistance of doctors, hospitals, and supporting staff. We are far better off with our "unnatural" hospital or birthing center deliveries in terms of survival and decreased complications. The point is that we must not believe that everything we do in hospitals and birthing centers is necessary. What we do is provide a safety net in the event of a problem, but delivery is still a simple, natural act.

Delivering a baby in the hospital is similar to buying life insurance. I purchase life insurance to help my family if I should die. I really do not want to cash in my life insurance policy. I much prefer living. If I go on living, I do not care that I spent money on the insurance.

Similarly, mothers today deliver babies in hospitals to cover the possibility that a problem might arise in childbirth. No one wants to have a problem, but if one arises, hospital personnel are better equipped to handle it. In fact, most pregnant mothers have normal deliveries, and most delivered newborns are normal babies.

You will be delighted to have a normal baby and realize, when childbirth is completed, that the hospital support was comforting but not necessary. You will not care if your money was spent on the hospital if you have a fine, normal baby; you will be grateful to be hospitalized if you or your baby should need attention for a problem. Certainly, your recovery will be more pleasant and supported than our ancestors.

Nothing New Under the Sun

For womankind, childbirth is not new. Every new mother should trust her feelings and be confident that she can handle this situation just as her ancestors did. While it is much safer and more comfortable to deliver in a hospital or birthing center, sometimes our technologies and economic pressures go too far.

The Tony Award-winning Delivery: I Don't Think So

During my career, I have witnessed interventions to make birthing more comfortable. For a while, the use of scopolamine was very popular. Scopolamine is a drug that creates total amnesia in patients but leaves them able to talk and be aware. Many people know it as truth serum since, under its influence, people will talk and reveal secrets and yet not remember they did so. The delivering mother was so spaced-out that she recalled absolutely nothing about the delivery. Some women seemed to love the idea of waking up after delivering a baby and have no recollection of any pain. The sad part was that the mother-to-be was taken out of the picture. She could not tell you where her pain was, and medical support staff lost valuable input from the mother as to the possibility of a potential problem. Not recalling the birth pain may have been a benefit to the mother, but by taking the mother out of the picture, it could lead to problems for the obstetrician.

I have also witnessed interventions to make delivery more predictable and "on time." Several years ago, forceps delivery was popular. Rather than wait for the delivery to occur naturally, forceps could be applied to engage a baby's head and pull it out of the birth canal sooner. This could shorten the period of painful labor for the mother. Unfortunately, the baby often came out with facial trauma or even a fracture. Today, forceps-assisted deliveries are used only when absolutely necessary rather than as a measure of convenience.

Within the last several years, the latest new intervention has been the performance of an elective caesarean section for first pregnancies. With elective C-sections, mothers need not go through labor, and the time and date of delivery can be set definitively. These designer deliveries have their drawbacks. The most significant problem is that we do not know when a given pregnancy has reached term. Full-term babies range from thirty-seven to forty-one weeks. We know that some infants require a longer gestation than others. Baring any problems in the mother that might suggest the need for an early delivery, it makes sense to allow a baby to mature until the moment that nature says it's time to deliver. That proper moment is the onset of labor and not a moment chosen at the convenience of the mother and obstetrician. More often than not, nature comes up with better timing as to the maturity of the fetus than the clinician.

Nancy's Story: Childbirth Doesn't Always Happen as Planned

With our first baby, I began labor at nine o'clock in the evening. Already overdue by almost a week, I dreaded any more telephone calls from family and friends.

"You're still home? Why haven't you delivered? Why hasn't that baby entered the world by now? Are you trying to induce labor? Try spicy food."

Desperate, I listened to the latter advice and ate very spicy Indian food for dinner. That trick worked! Within two hours, I was in labor.

But don't jump to conclusions. After a few hours in the hospital, during which my contractions were timed by nurses, the obstetrical resident sent me home.

"You are not in labor. Your contractions are not intense enough. Go home and rest."

Rest was impossible. The contractions kept coming. While the contractions may not have been intense enough for the resident to pronounce as labor, they were certainly intense enough for me. Finally, as soon as my obstetrician's office opened, I called and was given an appointment that morning for an examination by Dr. Mezer, who decided that I was definitely in labor, so we returned to the hospital by midday. After many more contractions, my labor had not progressed, and I began to have the sinking feeling that I would be a failure at childbirth. An x-ray clarified the situation. My pelvic opening was too small for my baby's head. Dr. Mezer recommended an emergency caesarean section.

My feelings of failure and disappointment were intense. We had attended two birthing classes, I had read several books about childbirth and breast-feeding, and I felt very ready. In my classes and in the books I had read, C-sections received barely a mention, and I had not even once thought that I would face that situation. But now, the only alternative was stark: our baby could not enter the birth canal and would die if not delivered by surgery.

Having had twenty-one hours of contractions, I was too exhausted to continue my focus on the process of childbirth; I was relieved that my baby would finally be delivered. When I woke the next day, I was acutely aware of both the pain from the surgery and of the regret that I had not been able to deliver vaginally. Friends who had also delivered their babies by caesarean section shared their disappointment and regret.

My sister reminded me of a story that our father had told us years earlier. A poor farmer ached to buy a pair of beautiful shoes because the ones that he had were ragged. One day, after staring longingly into the window of a fine leather shop, he turned to see an unusual passerby in a wheelchair: a man who had no feet. Instantly, the farmer recognized his mistake; instead of daydreaming about new shoes, he returned home to repair and polish his old ones. He then placed them lovingly on his feet, realizing how privileged he was that he still had feet.

The lesson was clear: focus on the positive and cheer about what was fortunate in my situation. I had a healthy baby girl, I would shortly heal from the C-section, and I could be upbeat about my circumstances.

Obstetric Technologies: Pros and Cons

Today, we have the ability to induce labor and schedule caesarean sections. Scheduling deliveries makes good medical sense for a repeat C-section or a primary C-section where the baby's position in the uterus warrants this type of delivery. A planned caesarean section decreases the risk factors for the infant and the mother. However, it makes little sense to use pitocin to speed up delivery or rush to a caesarean section when convenience is the only issue. Ideally, the less intervention in the natural process of childbirth, the better off both infant and mother will be. Just because we have the technologies to intervene does not mean they are always necessary or appropriate. The bottom line is that you are going to a hospital to cover that rare instance when everything does not go well. Until there is a problem, there are no reasons for interventions. You are in the hospital with the hope and likelihood that you don't have to be there in the first place.

- Nature works on a slow track. It takes months to make a baby and many hours of labor to deliver it. There is no good reason to rush these processes.

- You have a three- to four-day safety margin built in before feeding your newborn becomes the focus of your attention. As noted above, natural things take time.

- Hospitals and birthing centers provide a safe environment to cover the unexpected and rare problems and situations. Keep in mind that rare things only occur rarely.

Dan and I found that the process of writing a book can be very stressful. Fortunately, we did have some moments of laughter, especially when writing the limericks that grace (!) a few of the chapters, and also when we looked into practices involving pla-centas. We were on a long car trip when I asked Dan, "When did women stop eating their placentas? I cannot picture that Queen Victoria ate hers!" We both chuckled at this thought and Dan said he would do some research.

That research consisted of asking his former student, Dr. Anjali Kaimal, then an obstretrics resident at the Brigham & Women's Hospital, what she knew of the history of placenta-eating. Soon Anjali, a master googler, came back with an e-mail entitled "Yum!"

Placentophagia, or eating the placenta, is still practiced in underdeveloped parts of the world (which we knew). But, it is also practiced in the developed world, especially judging by the number of recipes that can be found on the web. And we learned that a placenta is really the only animal organ that vegans can eat (since no animal is killed to obtain it). Thereafter, the mention of braised placenta, roasted placenta, or pla-centa primavera sent us, and our friends with whom we shared this information, into gales of laughter. My apologies to serious placenta eaters.

3

The First Ten Minutes

A sperm meets an egg deep inside
For nine months cells grow and divide
Then you push and you shove
In a labor of love,
Take a break and lie side by side.

Admire baby's fingers and toes,
As you gaze, your pride just grows and grows.
But perfect she's not,
Homo Sapiens's her lot,
Enjoy and forget any woes.

The journey from pregnancy to delivery resembles a roller-coaster ride. During the first long, slow, uphill climb, anticipation builds; then, the roller-coaster crescendos into that first rapid descent down a long super steep incline. The last few weeks of pregnancy that ends in labor is like that long climb uphill; you are eager to deliver but may feel some trepidation about the delivery, which, when it happens, mimics that exciting finish. But unlike the roller-coaster ride, the time for relaxation is not over the first moment after the baby is delivered. In those first five to ten minutes, newborns have serious work awaiting them.

Predicting a Birth Date Is Like Predicting the Weather

A full-term baby has a gestational age of thirty-seven to forty-one weeks, a full four-week period. We cannot, despite our modern technology, predict the birth date of a baby more precisely than that. In fact, we do not know what factor in nature decides when labor will begin. The onset of labor most likely relates to a combination of many factors. Foremost among these is the ability of the placenta to continue supplying adequate calories, nutrients, and oxygen to the growing fetus. When the placenta begins to calcify and its vessels are not performing at maximum, some signals must pass between the mother and growing fetus that urge the infant to begin using her own stored caloric sources for energy.

Where's the Fat?

Almost all newborns, including all three of my own, look as if they have just finished a crash course in weight loss. Their cheeks appear well filled out, but their skinny chicken legs have elephantlike flabby skin. The important question is not where the beef is, but where the fat is. When the calories delivered to the fetus by the placenta no longer meet the growth demands of the infant, the baby begins to burn up the fatty stores in the legs. The triggers are set for an exit from the uterus.

The uterine environment, in some ways, is akin to the environment on a spaceship. Supplies are perfectly adequate for a defined period, but a landing becomes necessary when that period has elapsed. Birth is that landing, but unlike our astronaut who is returning to a well-known environment, a newborn is about to experience a radical change when she emerges from the womb into our world. For the first time, the newborn's respiratory, cardiac, vascular, endocrine, gastrointestinal, and neurological functions all have to take over in a period of seconds and adapt to this new environment. After thirty years as a pediatrician, I still marvel at a newborn baby. All my pediatrician and neonatologist friends agree; we are awestruck by what is happening in those first tense moments after a baby leaves the security of the womb.

So Much to Accomplish but So Little Time

Visualize what occurs in those first few moments. Babies emerge from a womb where the temperature is 100 to 101 degrees farenheit into a room temperature of 70 degrees farenheit. They need to quickly constrict the blood vessels in the skin to conserve heat. They must shift the fluid that fills their lungs so that they can inhale oxygen from the air.

A Breath of Fresh Air

Until delivery, oxygenated blood came directly to the infant through the placenta. Suddenly, babies must get their oxygen from the air. The newborns' first attempts at inhaling are critical for the transition to life on earth for two reasons. First, with inhalation, newborns push the fluid from their lungs into their bodies, giving themselves the needed hydration to sustain and support their circulation for the first several days of life. During those few days, mothers are able to clear lactation-blocking hormones from their systems and begin to make milk, and babies need that time to figure out how to suck.

Whereas in utero passive fetuses receive food through the placenta, active infants must obtain new calories from an outside source. In the interim before newborns realize how to suck and before mothers can make breast milk, infants burn some saved calorie stores from fat deposits and muscles. The burning of these calories accounts for part of the 10 percent weight loss that babies experience during the first few days. Nature decided that newborns do not have to accomplish the full transition to life outside the uterus on the first or second day of life. Feeding does not head the agenda in these first moments. The first inhalations provide a backup fluid supply, and the fats and muscles are a backup food supply.

Will Her Lungs Expand?

Secondly, inhaling expands the lung tissues to allow the exchange of oxygen between the atmosphere and infant's circulatory system. To continue the space analogy, without lung expansion, we face a mission-critical situation. For the first few minutes after an infant is born, those assisting in the delivery experience a haunting silence, like the silence of those in mission control who waited for Apollo 13 to come back into communication with Earth. When voice contact resumed, NASA staff were elated, just as Nancy and I and every other new parent feel pure elation when we finally hear a cry from the baby. As a pediatric resident in the delivery room, my heart raced as we waited for that same cry. I was trained to provide minimal support while a baby undergoes transition through the conversion process to extrauterine life.

A Systems Check

And while we perform our roles as participants in this birth, the infant is the one who does the majority of the work. During these same moments of lung expansion, volume absorption, and oxygen exchange, the cardiovascular system of the infant is radically changing as well. Until the umbilical cord is cut, the circulatory system of the infant takes a unique route. Since the blood gets oxygen from the mother's breathing and the baby's lungs are filled with fluid, blood doesn't circulate through the infant's lungs. Very little blood flows into the pulmonary artery to the baby's lungs and back to the baby's heart. Indeed, there are holes between the chambers of the baby's heart to let the blood bypass the baby's lungs. The function of a special artery called the ductus arteriosus is to avoid blood flow to the lungs. Just as the lungs expand and change into a functional oxygenator in those first few minutes, so too the heart of the baby, and the direction of blood flow also changes dramatically upon arrival on planet Earth. The baby has made another major adjustment from in-utero life to life on earth. And this amazing transformation is accomplished without any assistance from the adults.

Breathing or Feeding—Which Shall It Be?

Several pediatric advice books stress the importance of the bonding of a new mother and her infant, bonding that supposedly begins at the moment of birth. I don't think so! The baby has a great deal more on its agenda in these first minutes than bonding and breast-feeding. If the respiratory and cardiovascular systems do not successfully make the adjustments noted above, there will be no bonding and no breast-feeding. The current focus on bonding and breast-feeding in the first few minutes sets up false expectations for new mothers about the first minutes after delivery. We are in a mad rush to move well-programmed natural processes along at an accelerated tempo rather than to trust in nature.

Likewise, our cave women ancestor was not about to bond and breast-feed either. She was dehydrated, bleeding profusely, and exhausted. In addition, she was in the throws of continuing contractions, and she had to deliver the placenta. Not surprisingly, the transition to extrauterine life had to be left to the newborn infant to accomplish on its own. The new mother has her own major transitions to keep her very busy. Her cardiovascular system has to accommodate a sudden, major blood loss on top of a prolonged period of dehydration and volume loss.

Many People but Little Work to Do

Among the "unnatural" aspects of today's childbirth is that new mothers are well hydrated, free of pain, and very much alert and aware of what is going on. In the delivery room, a new father, an obstetrician or midwife, a pediatrician, an anesthesiologist, and various nursing personnel assist the mother at the moment of delivery. But unless the infant or mother has a problem, all of these people have very little to do. The newborn infant is going to make the transition to life all by itself.

Nancy's Story: "Please, please, please, bring my baby to me."

With our third child, I underwent amniocentesis, a procedure during which a physician extracts fluid from the amniotic sac of a pregnant woman and then microscopically examines the chromosomes found in that fluid. The fluid should contain both maternal and fetal chromosomes. If only female chromosomes are found, the result is ambiguous because the captured chromosomes may have been only the mother's. If male chromosomes are present, however, the baby must be male because his mother doesn't have male chromosomes of her own. In my case, I was told that I was having a boy. "Think blue," said the geneticist who analyzed the amniotic fluid.

That news was disappointing to me. We had two children, one girl and one boy. My relationship with my sister was very strong, and I wanted another girl so that my daughters would have a chance to have such a close relationship. Of course, it is true that once the baby comes, one loves him or her, whatever the case may be.

We selected boy names, called our family and friends, and told our young children. I bought baby clothes appropriate for a boy. Since I was having my third C-section, we not only knew the sex of the baby, but also his birthday as well.

In the delivery room, the nursing staff had filled out the birth certificate as "Male Heller." The anesthesiologist gave me an epidural anesthesia to numb my abdomen and legs but not my upper torso and head. I was awake and alert when Dr. Mezer performed the C-section and extracted the baby from my womb. In a matter-of-fact and low-key manner, he said, "Oh, it's a girl."

"A girl!" I screamed. "That's <u>impossible</u>; there must be another baby in there!"

He accepted my logic and started to probe in my uterus. Holding my breath as I waited for the answer, I could feel the pushing and shoving of the probe but had no pain. I looked at my husband, who stood next to me. He was grinning as if this was the result we had expected all along.

"No, she's the only one," Dr. Mezer said in a stunned tone of voice as he realized the implications.

"Let me see her!" I shouted as I turned my attention to our baby.

But no one brought her to me. Everyone was silent. During my two previous deliveries, a nurse had talked in reassuring tones to let me know what was happening. But no one was talking this time. My fears were mounting.

"What's taking so long? I want to see her," I implored.

More than 25 years later, I still have a clear recollection of those several minutes. At the time, I felt that I waited an eternity to see my baby girl, who was supposed to be a baby boy. But then, an understanding of what my baby was accomplishing was not on my radar screen. Despite the fact that she was our third child, I had no idea of the feats that she engaged in, that she was in a fragile period of coming to life, and that such a period is several minutes longer than any book or movie had led me to believe. In books and movies, an infant is given a pat on the bottom and begins to cry. I did not appreciate that the cry occurs at the beginning of the transitional phase.

In hindsight, the medical and support personnel in that room must have been holding their breaths as they waited for our baby to breathe on her own. Since she was supposed to be male, perhaps they wondered if she was deformed or abnormal in some way. After what seemed like an interminable wait, a nurse brought her to me for a confirmatory view. She was definitely a girl! And subsequent chromosomal testing proved it.

What neither they nor we knew then was that a simple laboratory error labeled our baby as a boy. Marissa thought that her diligent wishing to the blue fairy for a sister had changed our baby from a boy to a girl. She convinced Matt of this fact, and he was upset that the blue fairy favored his older sister and granted her wish! Dan's job was to convince both of them that the blue fairy had had nothing to do with this apparent intrauterine sex transformation.

What's Not for Dinner?

At the five-minute mark of life, a major change transpires in the atmosphere of the delivery room. The obstetrician, the pediatrician, the new parents, and all others produce a united sigh of relief. The infant has landed and made the transition to earthly life. <u>Now</u> is the time to hold and cuddle and share body warmth with your new baby. Both mother and baby are quite exhausted at this moment. Many pediatricians, supported by the hospital's clinical practice guidelines, urge mothers to nurse at this moment. Nursing at this emotionally charged time is not necessary. The baby had just experienced very complex and tiring transitions; the last question on his/her mind is what's for dinner.

Let's Skip Dinner: I've Got a Lot to Do Today

With respiratory and cardiovascular systems only newly functioning, one can wait for one to three before testing the gastrointestinal system. In fact, the neurological system is the next to begin reacting.

Our newborn has been cramped up inside a very small container and surrounded by fluid for nine months. For the first time, she is receiving some stimuli through her fingers and toes. Her skin is being touched for the first time and is sending a multitude of impulses and information to her brain. Her ears and eyes are also receiving new messages. The sensory inputs suddenly impacting this new human being are colossal. On the other hand, she has a very immature central nervous system, which is easily overwhelmed by these inputs. The best approach at this moment is to introduce calmness and tenderness. Rather than forcing a nipple into the baby's mouth and saying, "Eat, eat, eat," our strategy should be to minimize inputs. Our modern fast-paced lifestyle does not have to begin on the sixth minute of life. I urge you to make the next hours peaceful and serene. In truth, since neither the mother nor the infant needs to do much of anything for the next three days, this is the perfect time to linger without the stress of rushing to the next step.

The chapters on childbirth and breast-feeding should make it perfectly clear that after the infant has survived the transition to extrauterine life and after the mother has survived the process of childbirth, both are entitled to a few days of relaxation. Indeed, that period of rest was built into nature's scheme.

But the rest period has been seriously compromised because of economic and legal pressures rather than medical necessity. The economic drive is to discharge the mother and the baby from the hospital as quickly as possible. The legal drive is to protect the hospital from any liability incurred by this economic push.

Great Job: Why Not Take a Few Days Off?

As the proud new owner of a baby, parents have three full days just to admire the beauty of their newborn and discover how perfect he or she is. Nancy and I will never forget the first moments after Marissa was born. When the obstetrician extracted Marissa from Nancy's womb, he announced that the baby was a girl, and she was perfect. He immediately handed her to me, as the pediatrician, to do the initial newborn assessment.

That assessment consists of assigning an APGAR score to the infant at one minute of life and at five minutes of life. This scoring system, named after Dr. Virginia Apgar, established a quick method of appraisal of the newborn infant. The system serves as a means of separating those newborns who might have a significant anatomic or physiologic defect at birth from those who are likely normal. Each APGAR score rates the baby on five easily observed or measured criteria.

Included are the respiratory rate, the heart rate, the skin color, the infant's reflex irritability or cry, and the infant's muscular tone. Each criterion is assigned a rating of zero, one, or two. Since the scoring is based on five criteria, each with the potential to earn a score of two, the best score is a ten; and the worst is obviously a zero. Rarely do babies attain a score of ten; their color is almost always not quite pink, and mucus disrupts their respirations. Usually, the scores are seven at one minute and increase after five minutes to nine. However, scores below six or scores that decrease from one minute to five minutes suggest that there may be a problem.

Perfection Is in the Eye of the Beholder

When Marissa was handed to me, as a pediatrician, to perform the initial assessment, the only scoring that I did was counting her fingers and toes and confirming that she had two eyes, a nose, and a mouth. I never checked her heart rate or respirations or tone or color. Our obstetrician asked me after five minutes what the APGAR scores were. I quickly responded that the APGAR scores were ten at one minute and ten at five minutes. When he stared at me with a doubtful expression, I replied that I had based my scoring on the baby's fingers and toes rather than the usual criteria. Of course, I was thrilled that she looked normal. As I told my relatives and friends about my "perfect" ten-and-ten-APGAR baby, I realized that I shared the same desire of every new parent, the desire for a perfect baby. I have met with pre-adoptive parents who are particularly open in their desire to have a child with no defects. But there are no perfect babies. I can find something "wrong" with almost every newborn I examine. Most of these imperfections are of no consequence; in fact, they remind us that a newborn is the result of an incredible series of events.

Every Baby Is a Lottery Winner

In a sense, every new baby is a one-in-four-hundred-million shot, a definite lottery winner. The fact is that one sperm out of two to four hundred million sperms finds an egg very transiently at a point where it can be fertilized. This one egg and one sperm then form a single cell that splits millions of times and results in the creation of liver tissue, heart tissue, muscle tissue, bones, tendons, brains, skins, eyes, blood cells, and so on. Within six to eight weeks of that initial joining of an egg and a sperm, almost every major organ system is defined in the fetus. Most new moms are not even aware of their pregnancy by the time that these major developments have occurred. Pregnant women begin to monitor their diets, control any bad habits like smoking and alcohol use, and avoid any toxins after the differentiation of all the organ systems are well under way. Considering that conception faces many obstacles, the fact that most babies are nearly perfect at birth is quite astonishing. Not surprisingly, this process does not always happen according to nature's design.

On the Other Hand, Maybe She Is Not So Perfect

Marissa was not as perfect at birth as I had initially presumed. Within a few hours, I began to wonder why her chin protruded and her eyelids were so swollen. She had greasy white material behind her ears and over her scalp. Her skin was blotchy and had many pimples that seemed to come and go. Her legs seemed bowed, and one foot turned in. And all that was just on the outside. What we did not know then, and discovered three years later, was that her kidneys were not draining properly. These design defects were all resolved over time. She had external dings and dents, findings that are actually normal in all babies, and her internal design defects were fixable surgically. The point is that neither she nor any newborn is "perfect." What I learned from the birth of my own daughter and from caring for so many others is that, while not perfect, most newborns come well equipped by Mother Nature to survive and thrive. Perfection is a goal rather than a reality. Over thousands of years, we are slowly evolving as a species, and we are only a moment in that evolution. We are improving and adapting but never achieving perfection. Mother Nature provides us with newborns who have the right parts in the right place most of the time.

- Labor and delivery is hard work, and a mother deserves a break.

- Babies performed hard work at their deliveries, and they deserve a break as well.

- The first ten minutes of life represent enormous transitions for the baby.

- Moms need time to adjust to and settle into their new role.

- Babies need time to adjust to and settle into their new role.

- No delivery is perfect; no baby is perfect.

Dr. Jeffrey Katz, an obstetrician, wrote,

Recently, while waiting for the elevator first thing in the morning, Dan seemed unusually enthusiastic. After exchanging the usual pleasantries, I asked him why he seemed so happy. He then explained that he had just taken care of a newborn baby and "what could be better"! The delight he took in doing his work was certainly contagious. This simple memory brings a smile to my face.

4

Up Close and Personal

The first day of life is a time to sit back, relax, and catch one's breath. The mother and the baby have endured enormous physiologic changes and have both survived. The roller-coaster has stopped; with somewhat shaky legs, you can take the time to reassess and reassure yourself that all your body parts are still intact. Sometime during this first twenty-four hours, your pediatrician will examine the baby. I personally love the circumstance when the infant is in the mother's room; I can sit on the bed and identify for new parents all the details of their newborn. After all, everyone in the family has been waiting for nine months for this brand-new baby. Let's pick up the owner's manual for information about the functions of various parts and about what extras may be included in this brand-new model XX or XY human. Oops, no owner's manual came with delivery.

The next best thing is to explain to you what a pediatrician looks for and what information that specific examination findings reveal about the baby. As mentioned before, no newborn is perfect. Some imperfections disappear with time, some will not but are of no consequence, and some are possible signs of underlying problems. Let's take a look at a "normal" newborn from head to toe.

Owners Manual for Twenty-first Century Babies

The Head Does the Work

The newly delivered head is not a pretty sight. Imagine that your head was used for several hours as a battering ram to break down the gates of a medieval castle. That is exactly what the head of your newborn was used for during labor. Her head pushed through the narrow cervix with the help of uterine muscles contracting against her body. The result of this constant pressing and pushing is that her head takes on the shape of the tight uterine opening and resembles a cone. The top of her head literally appears to be peaked.

29

The appearance of her head is also affected by a second factor; the head is the largest and least compressible part of any newborn's body. After the head is pushed through the cervix, delivering the rest of the infant's body is straightforward. In order to facilitate delivery of the head and protect it, nature designed a clever system in which the skull bones themselves are not fused together. The frontal, parietal, and occipital bones are in the form of independent bony plates, which have the ability to slide over one another. This ability allows the skull to be squashed a bit during delivery so that it can slide through the cervix, but the trade-off is that the baby arrives with a rather asymmetric-shaped skull. At birth, any newborn's skull viewed from almost any angle will not be symmetrical and ideally shaped like a classic Greek statue. It may take days to weeks for the true shape of the skull to manifest itself.

In addition to asymmetry, the skull has a very inconsistent texture with hard, bony parts that have diamond-shaped soft spots in between; frequently, there may also be a large soft circular bump. The soft spots are called fontanelles, suture lines that occur at those points where the bony plates come close together. At these soft spots, the non-fused bones can slide up to and over one another to compress during delivery. The large soft circular bump, on the other hand, is a cephalohematoma. Remember that for hours the skull was used as a ramrod, and the area of swelling is the part that took the most direct contact. That bump is filled with fluid and blood and may take weeks to flatten out and disappear. Rarely, a cephalohematoma represents a fracture of the skull bone that occurred during delivery, but these hardly ever present a problem and flatten with time.

A Face Only a Mother Could Love

First, the Eyes

In the nursery, doctors and nurses enjoy looking at the faces of babies despite the fact that those faces are not usually pretty. Perhaps the marvel of reproduction has all of us light-headed and proud. On close inspection, observe that babies have swollen eyelids as a consequence of the pushing and the application of a protective antibiotic ointment. Their lids are full of edema fluid, making it hard to see the eyeball itself. If the baby is able to open its eyes, we frequently notice bright blood red hemorrhages in the whites of the eyes. Again, this is due to the trauma of the delivery. The eyes themselves are crossed, giving the infant a cockeyed look, which is perfectly normal and can continue for as many as eight weeks. We cannot ascertain how well the eyes work at this early stage, but a pediatrician can test for a "red reflex." The subject of flash photography often has "red eyes." A light directed to the newborn's eyes will bring out this reflex to confirm that no cataract is blocking the light and that the infant has a retina. The retina functions as a screen to accept light and color, which the retina then converts into information that can enter the nervous system and be interpreted by the brain.

Next, the Nose

Most noses are relatively small and squashed; they face either to the right or the left. The nostrils are not equal in size and are also small and narrow, which means that a tiny quantity of mucus can sound like an enormous amount.

Ears and Mouth

Asymmetry in the human face is present not only at birth but at all ages and may be more noticeable in the ears and the mouth. The ears are frequently folded down or over and look very strange. In large part, this is due to the fact that the cartilage is not yet developed in the newborn's ears. Please be assured that, if folded, the ears will flatten out with time.

Frequently, babies appear to have two mouths; their chins are so indented as to resemble another orifice. Nancy's sister, Susan, was convinced that Marissa had two mouths; she practically accused me of begetting the most unusual baby. But these concerns disappear; indeed, what you first see in the face of your newborn is not what you will eventually see in relation to ears, noses, and mouths.

Rarely, a baby will have a cleft lip on one or both sides of the face and even extending up into the nasal cavity. Physical abnormalities on the face are, understandably, the most upsetting to new parents than any other abnormality. I have the advantage of having seen these deformities before and know that, with plastic surgery, they virtually disappear. But for parents who see such abnormalities for the first time, it is hard to imagine anything beautiful emerging from this beginning. A pediatrician and specialists should get involved early on and walk parents through the return to normalcy.

Another less common facial abnormality is a pre-auricular skin tag. A small nubbin of tissue in front of the ear, this skin tag is usually a mere cosmetic problem and is easily corrected by a plastic surgeon. On occasion, however, such a skin tag may have clinical significance since it is sometimes associated with hearing loss.

Today, with or without skin tags, newborns are routinely screened for hearing in many hospitals during the first forty-eight hours.

Red Marks: Will They Ever Disappear?

The head and face usually have some marks. The most common are flat red or purplish markings commonly called stork bites and angel kisses. According to folklore, the marks are formed when an angel kisses the baby on the face before giving her to the stork for delivery. Stork bites are located at the nape of the neck at the base of the skull, and angel kisses are found on the eyelids, forehead, and nose. Capillary hemangioma is the medical name for these markings. Capillary refers to small caliber blood vessels. *Hemangio* means "blood vessel," and *oma* means "tumor." Despite the fact that the word *tumor* is used, such hemangiomas are totally benign and disappear over the first three years of life with no treatment.

Far less common are "port wine stains." These areas of deep purple discoloration cover larger areas and are sometimes associated with underlying neurologic disorders, which is why pediatricians pay closer attention to these marks. In years past, such "stains" were permanent; but with today's laser technologies, they can be removed.

Babies Have Acne Too

Let's not forget "baby acne," which almost all newborns will have at delivery or will develop during the first week. Hormones are rapidly changing in the baby once the umbilical cord is tied off, and when hormones change, acne-like lesions appear. In fact, this period of hormonal readjustment occurs over the first eight to twelve weeks, which is why a baby's skin is not usually unblemished until almost three months of age. That beautiful baby soft skin we see and hear about in commercials is not present at birth but will appear by three months.

What Happened to the Neck?

I always have fun with the fact that most children look as if they are born with at least two chins but no neck. A newborn's head and chest are big; the head has been squashed down in the limited space of the uterus. As a result, a neck is not really apparent. Very importantly, your pediatrician will stretch the chin up to look at the crunched neck area. Very rarely, the neck has little slits on either side or some bony material that are remnants of primitive gill slits present during fetal life. If such remnants are present, surgical intervention may be necessary.

Also note that the head and neck are usually turned to one side or the other. Indeed, in many infants, the head will not move all the way to one side. This is a condition called congenital torticollis or wry neck. In the fetal position in utero, the head is usually turned to one side or the other for a substantial period of the gestation. Therefore, the neck muscles on one side will be shorter and tighter than the muscles on the other side. These muscles will slowly loosen up, and mobility of the neck will increase with time.

Chests: All Babies Have Breasts

For new parents, another disconcerting feature of a newborn is the bumps behind the baby nipples. Whether boy or girl, that baby has spent the last nine months inside a mother. In that environment, the fetus has been steadily exposed to normal adult levels of female hormones. Therefore, in both sexes, breast tissue has been stimulated by these hormones. In fact, if nursed, the baby will get lactating hormones through the breast milk; and this, combined with their levels of female hormones, will cause them to secrete milk by one to two weeks of age. Such phenomenon is entirely normal; both breast tissue and milk will decrease over time as the infant slowly loses those adult female hormones.

Abs: Outie versus Innie

As we all know, some babies end up with belly buttons that stick out; others have belly buttons that curve in. Please do not blame your obstetrician, who definitely does not control whether a baby has an outie or innie. The umbilical cord is cut after delivery and clamped off. No matter where that clamp is placed, whether one inch or one foot from the infant, the remaining piece of cord will dry up to a spot that nature established as the interphase of the infant circulation versus the maternal circulation. Thus, Mother Nature is to blame for an ugly belly button.

At birth, babies have very underdeveloped abdominal muscles, which make it impossible to figure out whether a particular baby will have an outie or innie. Babies' bellies are floppy because the abdominal rectus muscles are only about the width of a finger, running up and down the abdominal wall. Any structures along the sides of the abdomen or in the midline of the abdomen cannot be pulled in by tightening these tiny abdominal muscles. The maturation of the abdominal muscles occurs over several years; many belly buttons don't look as cute as a button for three years because they are not pulled in before that time.

Some infants have a defect in the abdominal wall, which allows an umbilical hernia to develop. Many of these are not problematic and will resolve as the abdominal muscles mature. In some instances, the umbilical hernia does require correction by a surgical procedure.

Finally, the chest and abdomen are the perfect place to spot all kinds of rashes. Generally called normal newborn rash, they include bumps like mosquito bites that seem to come and go within minutes and areas of redness that also are here today and gone tomorrow. The cause of these rashes can be internally driven as the newborn's microcirculatory system in the skin adjusts itself, causing increased or decreased blood flow to certain areas. The cause can also be externally driven as the baby's skin, after months of floating in amniotic fluid, is now in contact with an array of fabrics, cleansers, lotions, and potions. Almost all such rashes are benign and require no treatment.

Flip the Baby Over: Hair Today, Gone Tomorrow

Rashes similar to those on the chest and abdomen are common on the back as well.

In addition, the back has a monopoly on "Mongolian spots." Mongolian spots resemble big flat bruises over the buttocks and lower back and extend on to the thighs. Even though labeled as Mongolian, these spots are not related to mongolism or Down's syndrome, which is a chromosomal disorder, and they are not related to Mongolians as a race. These spots are common in infants whose family trees have roots around the Mediterranean basin. These spots need no treatment, and fortunately, they vanish with time, usually about five to six years.

A baby's back frequently has hair. Light hair, dark hair, fine hair, or coarse hair—all may show up on the back. The texture and color make no difference. My experience is that, over time, most of these hairs tend to tone down or recede. Some infants remain more hairy than others, but we have no method of predicting who will retain body hair.

Hair located at the crease in the midline of the lower back, just above the rectum, and in line with the lumbar-sacral spine may represent a problem. This place on human bodies is important to the development of the nervous system. As the embryo develops in utero, the spinal cord and vertebral bones are sealed off at the base of the spine. The overlying skin comes together over the nerves and bone, almost as if it was being zippered closed from the head down to the rectum. If the system does not close properly, significant problems may occur. Hair or abnormal dents, clefts, or creases in this lower spinal area are sometimes associated with neural tube defects. The worst of these problems is meningomyelocoele in which the spinal cord is not covered and the nerves do not work. Now that mothers take folic acid, we see less and less of this type of problem. Lesser degrees of injury can also occur and, at times, may not be apparent at all. Thus, abnormalities of the skin at the surface in this area may be a clue to abnormalities of the underlying structures. Therefore, midline tufts of hair, deep cavities, or sinus tracts in this location may be pursued by your pediatrician with an ultrasound to detect whether the underlying structures are normal.

Whether Boy or Girl: Well-endowed

We often hear such exclamations as "It's a boy!" or "It's a girl!" and "What an impressive boy or girl he or she is." As noted above, babies come from an intrauterine environment overflowing with high levels of hormones from both maternal and placental origins. These hormones stimulate tissues in the newborn baby's body of whatever gender.

In boys, the penis is usually large compared to the overall size of the infant. A secondary hormonal enhancing effect is the enlargement of the scrotal sack. As the effects of these hormones disappear between six to twelve months, the penis and scrotum actually decrease in size. Almost all parents, at the nine-month or one-year visit, are relieved to hear that the disappearance of their child's penis into the pubertal fat tissue is normal and that the penis shall someday rise again.

The scrotal sack, on the other hand, may be large due to a hernia or a hydrocele. A hernia is the result of the intestine sliding out of the abdomen through the inguinal ring and into the scrotal sack. Hernias in a newborn usually need to be repaired through an easy surgical procedure. A hydrocele, on the other hand, is simply fluid that is retained in the scrotal sack, and that fluid will usually reabsorb on its own.

In girls, uterine hormonal levels cause the enlargement of the labia on either side of the vagina as well as moistness of the vaginal mucosa. In many girls, the stimulating effect of these hormones is enough to cause the skin along the vaginal canal to overflow and actually hang out of the vagina as a mucous tissue. Over time, this tissue will recede back into the vaginal canal without any treatment.

Arms and Legs—Poorly Packaged

The uterus is not a very big place. Not surprisingly, once the space is filled with a big head, a large chest, and an abdomen, the arms, legs, hands, and feet have very little room. Mother Nature's solution is to shove the limbs in wherever they will fit. And shoved in they surely seem to be when I examine a baby. The arms and legs are in a flexed position and extending them fully always meets some resistance. Furthermore, the legs are folded over one another, causing them to be curved and bowed. The feet are then curled under even more. The extremities of newborns are definitely not perfect, but given time, they will usually unwind. Because of the degree of bowing, pediatricians have a difficult diagnostic challenge; some bowing and deformities are clinically significant and need treatment, while most do not. Usually, the best advice is to observe and reexamine, then observe and re-examine as the baby grows and the limbs stretch out.

This advice, however, is not applicable if the problem is in the hips or related to a clubfoot deformity. These problems can be diagnosed by your pediatrician, and treatment should begin sooner rather than later.

Hands, Feet, Fingers, and Toes—A Geneticist's Delight

When it comes to hands, feet, fingers, and toes, one could write an entire book. Geneticists linger on these parts and the face more than anything else because many bits of information are found in these places. The most obvious abnormality is having more than five digits for each extremity. Finding primitive makings of an an extra finger or toe is fairly common. Such extra digits are usually not fully developed and usually not functional. Years ago, pediatricians tied them off with a suture; the extra digit then fell off. More recently, plastic surgeons remove the extra digit.

Another common finding is the webbing of the skin between toes and, less commonly, between fingers. This webbing served a useful purpose when we were fish in the sea but is of no benefit now that we are land animals. If the webbing is significantly limiting, a surgeon can correct the problem for functional and cosmetic reasons.

On occasion, fingers or toes are longer or shorter than is common for the majority of people. This tends to be genetically programmed in some families but, sometimes, is a clue to an underlying metabolic or chromosomal abnormality. Such isolated "abnormalities," if alone, frequently have no significance at all. If, however, they occur with other abnormalities, they may indicate a problem. For example, most people have two major creases that cross in parallel the palm of the hand. A simian crease is the name given when there is only one crease across the palm. This simian crease is well-known to occur in children with Down's syndrome or mongolism. However, for children with this syndrome, the simian creases appear with other abnormalities in the eyes, ears, forehead, muscle tone, etc. Isolated simian creases are seen in doctors, lawyers, and teachers. Approximately one out of thirty normal people have a simian crease; if isolated with no other abnormalities, a simian crease is insignificant.

When I examine a newborn, I look for small details as well as observe the whole infant. Knowing that no baby is perfect, one must know which imperfections have significance and which can be ignored. Before new parents worry about features or issues that they have read or heard about, they should ask whether that feature or problem applies to their babies.

The Outside Was Examined, but What about the Inside?

The hardest work for a pediatrician is to check out all the pumps, filters, conduit tubing, electrical system, heating and ventilation equipment, and waste disposal units that come standard with your newborn. Medically, that means that I need to check the heart and lungs, pulses, and circulatory system. I feel inside a baby's abdomen for the liver and spleen and to feel for any abnormal masses. I make the baby go through a series of neurological maneuvers to check the intactness of her central nervous system. I fine no problem 99.9 percent of the time. Rarely do I ever find a problem that won't resolve on its own or be of no long-term consequence. Like all new parents, I can sit back and marvel at this creation of nature that is about as "perfect" as it can be. I leave the mother's room feeling good but not at all surprised that her baby is totally normal.

- **Most newborns are normal.**

- Most of a newborn's problems resolve with time or can be corrected medically or surgically.

- Squashed heads, asymmetrical faces, red marks, rashes, body hair, breast tissue, large groins, and curled limbs are all usual features of any newborn.

- Don't be afraid to ask your doctor about any feature of your newborn.

5

Breast-feeding, a Piece of Cake

Nursing can be really swell
Wrong advice makes it seem like such hell
Every dog, cat, and llama
Will feed from its mama
We're sure you can do it as well.

Breast-feeding: How Hard Can It Really Be?

I had a companion, Nina, who gave birth at home. She breast-fed all of her new-borns without any problems. She had not read one book about breast-feeding, had not seen one video, and never had a lactation consultant. Nina was our Siamese cat. It amazed me that the humans I was caring for needed so much input on the subject of breast-feeding when no other mammal on earth seemed to have a problem. How many cats, dogs, horses, cows, and monkeys choose to formula-feed? How many need my advice or that of a consultant in lactation? The answer is obvious. Someone has been playing "pediatricks" on us and ruining the natural bonding and satisfaction that nursing can engender.

Maternal Physiology 101: Getting Back to Basics

An understanding of breast-feeding is clearer if one understands the physiology behind it. A woman's body is miraculously designed to nurture a baby within it and then to nurture a baby outside it. The human body makes many changes to ensure that both roles will be successfully fulfilled. Among these changes is the growth of the placenta to intertwine the circulation of the fetus with that of the mother and the production of placental hormones to sustain a nine-month pregnancy. Hormones are chemicals that regulate body functions. One of the most important functions of these pregnancy hormones is to turn off the normal cycle of menstrual periods. This allows the uterus to provide a steady environment in which the fetus can grow. Obviously, if you continued having your period when you are pregnant, you could not sustain a normal gestation. For a period of thirty-seven to forty-one weeks, these hormones not only block the normal cycle of the uterus, but they also regulate the flow of blood and nutrients to the fetus.

An Interesting Hormone Side Effect: Surprise! You Can't Make Milk

Placental hormones present during pregnancy not only block menstrual periods, but they also block lactation hormones. Quite simply, you do not make milk during the time you are pregnant because of these placental hormones. The brain has cells that produce a lactating hormone. When released by the brain, lactating hormones travel through the blood to the glands in the breast and cause these glands to produce milk. Without lactating hormones, a woman's body cannot make milk. While placental hormones are in your body, the system involving lactating hormones is put on hold. Mother Nature seems to have figured out that you don't need the capacity to make milk until you have a baby.

Cave Woman Gives Birth: A Most Natural Act

In the chapter "Birth: A Most Unnatural Act Today," we imagined what childbirth was like for thousands of years. Let's return to our cave woman mother at the point of delivery and see how it relates to nursing a newborn. Remember that toward the end of the thirty-seven to forty-one weeks of pregnancy, our cave woman ancestor begins to feel ill. She gets intermittent abdominal cramps and loses her appetite for food and water. These symptoms worsen over the next twelve to twenty-four hours. This is labor, and "labor" it is. She becomes dehydrated, and her blood sugar levels are under stress. The pain at times may lead to moments of panic or unconsciousness. Finally, the blessed moment arrives as the cave mother pushes a newborn baby out of the uterine world and into our world.

Key Points to Remember

At the point of delivery, our new mother is obviously not in very good shape. She is dehydrated, low in blood sugar, nearly bleeding to death, and has NO milk. While modern medicine has improved a new mother's hydration and blood sugar level and minimized the loss of blood, it has not changed the physiology of a woman's body. Just like ten thousand years ago, today's breast-feeding mothers need three to seven days to clear lactation-blocking hormones from their bodies. Until these blocking hormones are gone, lactation cannot begin.

During this time, a new mother does have a bit of colostrum (a pre-milk fluid rich in antibodies). The amount of colostrum present can be consumed within a few minutes of a baby's sucking. Small amounts of sucking will also cause the release of oxytocins, which will help the uterus to contract and stop bleeding. But before she can produce real milk, our new mother has to clear the placental hormones. The only way to clear these blocking hormones is by peeing them out of her system. She must begin drinking and restoring her caloric intake. Nursing must take a backseat while the mother recovers from the birth process.

Breast-feeding Is Not on the Newborn's Agenda

Remember that when the baby comes into the real world, he breathes in air; this breathing of air causes the amniotic fluid in the lungs to be pushed across the pulmonary capillary bed and into the baby's circulation. This fluid represents an enormous volume of liquid that actually leaves the baby in an over-hydrated state. In fact, it will take three to four days for the baby to pee this extra fluid. The baby will lose weight (almost 10 percent of its birth weight), but much of this is actually just fluid weight. Until he pees off this fluid, he will hardly feel like sucking since, from the baby's point of view, he is over-hydrated. Nursing must take a backseat while the baby recovers from the birth process.

Also realize that the newborn baby is really a beehive of activity. He is taking over his respiratory, cardiovascular, endocrine, and neurological functions. There are sufficient supplies of fluid and nutrients to allow himr to put his gastrointestinal system on a back burner for three or four days. The last thing he needs is for a breast to be pushed into his face every two to three hours. He is getting enough inputs to integrate and does not need this extra distraction.

The Balance of Nature

Mother Nature has formulated a perfect harmony. It takes a new mother three to four days to make milk, and it takes an infant three to four days before becoming thirsty. Nature has provided a mother with a recovery period and a baby with a survival period. Other mammals, like our cave woman ancestors, know this intuitively. They need no advice or special devices. This breast-feeding thing must be a piece of cake if the entire animal kingdom can do it so easily.

How to Unsuccessfully Breast-feed Your Baby: Just Follow Today's Advice

And yet today, more and more mothers are frustrated by the nursing experience and feel incapable or inadequate for the task. I went to the hospital recently, and I examined nine newborns and talked to nine new mothers. All nine babies were from twelve to twenty hours old. Seven of the new mothers were in tears because the "nursing was not going well." They were frustrated and depressed on what should have been the happiest day of their lives. I heard comments such as "The baby won't latch on," "He won't wake up to feed," "My milk is not in," and "I'm ready to switch to the bottle because I don't think he is getting anything." The recurrent comment that really got to me was "I will *try* to nurse." I felt like crying and screaming at the same time. Why do new mothers today have these ideas, and why do they feel inadequate?

A Brief History of Breast-feeding

In the last ten years, hospitals have hired lactation consultants, bought breast pumps, and created more and more complex clinical practice guidelines to help mothers nurse better. How did something so easy become so complex? How did a basic mammalian function, breast-feeding, become an anxiety-producing function? Nature intended breast-feeding to be a way to nurture and sustain an infant. Instead, it seems that breast-feeding has become a way to nurture and sustain an industry. Today, lactation consultants are available in and out of hospitals, breast pumps are in every room by the baby's second day of life, formula is being presented to infants before mothers have a chance to make milk, and mothers feel like failures before they can possibly fail.

Slow and Steady Wins the Race

The answer to the question of why there is increasing pressure to nurse more quickly is not in medical literature, but rather in the policies of economic and legal departments. Thirty years ago, my first child was born. Marissa was kept in the nursery for the first twenty-four hours for "observation." Hospital guidelines suggested that newborns might throw up amniotic fluid or turn blue; the last thing we wanted to do was to begin nursing or feeding formula early. On the second day of life, Marissa was allowed out of the nursery, and Nancy was told to nurse for two minutes on a side every three to four hours and to increase this time by one minute for each of the nursing sessions on the next day and another minute for each of the nursing sessions of the day after that. By the fourth day, her milk came in, and Marissa was fine. Nancy was pleased since she was nursing well, and her nipples were only slightly chafed. Mothers at that time stayed in the hospital for four to seven days, and the pace was nice and slow.

Rooming in Becomes the Rage

Twenty years ago, the guidelines changed. Sara was born, and she did not have to stay for a day in the nursery. Hospitals realized that new moms did fine to have their babies with them. As to how often to feed and for how long, the rules were changed. Nancy was now told to feed for five to eight minutes on a side on the first day and increase to ten to fifteen minutes on the second day and twenty minutes by the third day. The idea was that early increased feeding time would bring the milk in more quickly. The result instead was that the milk still took four days to come in (some things don't change over ten thousand years). But now, Nancy had sore nipples and was in tears by the third day from the excessive sucking. Mothers were still allowed to stay in the hospital for three to seven days, and the pace was still relatively nice and slow.

Economic Crunch Time

More recently, managed care administrators decided to put some pressure on the system. Payors wanted vaginally delivered babies to go home by forty-eight hours and C-section deliveries to be home by day four. The doctors said fine since doctors always like a good challenge, and the hospital said fine since they could save money on "bed days." Mothers were even paid to leave early or were promised home visits to help them out. I think the problem came about when the hospital lawyers and quality assurance people said, "How can we be sure the nursing is going well at forty-eight hours, and how can we be sure the baby is OK?"

The answer should have been "We can't."

Nursing cannot be going well on day two since nursing is not happening at all on day two. Like it or not, we cannot make the breast milk come in more quickly than nature intended. Just as they did ten thousand years ago, mothers today still have to clear the lactation-blocking hormones in their bodies. It is unreasonable to ask a mother on day two or three how her nursing is going since it hasn't happened yet. Infants are still well hydrated and need nothing.

However, instead of saying "we can't," the hospitals and doctors decided to say "we can." Unfortunately, the clinical practice guidelines that the doctors and lactation consultants developed may meet the needs of the hospital lawyers and the payors (insurance companies), but they certainly do not meet the needs of the new mother and her baby.

Lactation consultants, on day one, tell mothers how to hold the baby, attempt to force a sleepy, over-hydrated infant to suck, and, when the baby doesn't suck, attach a machine to a mother's breasts to suck in place of the infant. Newborns now are introduced to formula feedings in the first two days of life to cover the economic pressures for early discharge. How unnatural can you get? But whether this is natural or unnatural makes very little difference.

Medical Crunch Time: Jaundice, Breast Milk, and Early Discharge

It is a well-established fact that bilirubin, a breakdown product of blood, is removed from the body when the liver and gastrointestinal system are functioning in their digestive and excretory capacities. Up to the moment of birth, bilirubin is rerouted through the umbilical cord and back to the mother to be excreted by her. After the umbilical cord is cut, the baby assumes the function of bilirubin excretion. A newborn's liver and gastrointestinal system are not immediately capable of assuming this task. Bilirubin begins to rise in all babies over the first few days of life. In most cases, the newborns' livers, by the third to fifth day of life, become mature enough to process bilirubin. Sometimes, the level of bilirubin becomes excessive; the newborn becomes jaundiced and may require treatment. Newborns with severely elevated bilirubin levels may suffer brain damage.

With the push for early discharge, the number of instances of undetected jaundice in newborn babies has increased. Jaundice frequently does not appear until day three, four, or five of life. Years ago, jaundice in babies was noticed by clinicians because newborns were still in the hospital. Now, many babies, discharged from hospitals forty-eight hours after birth, are not evaluated by clinicians until those babies are a week or two of age. As a result of early discharge and delayed follow-up, jaundice may be undetected and may reach more toxic levels than it would have if it had been observed earlier. This rise in clinically significant jaundice is not a consequence of inadequate breast-feeding but rather a direct consequence of early discharge coupled with delayed diagnosis. The best way to evaluate a newborn's jaundice risk is for providers to examine babies on day three to five of life as part of a routine discharge follow-up visit. The American Academy of Pediatrics now recommends this as well.

You Cannot Beat Mother Nature

This plan to overcome the forces of nature and induce mothers to lactate quickly has not worked. Instead, we have mothers sitting in rooms with breast pumps sucking at their breasts instead of infants. We have mothers feeling frustrated and inadequate. It's time to stop the madness. Some natural processes are better left on their own. We ought to allow mothers and babies to begin the nursing process slowly and refocus our support on making nursing a piece of cake.

Nancy's Story: Breast-feeding Was a Piece of Cake

Today, I hear horror stories of women who give up nursing after forty-eight hours. Luckily, for those of us who gave birth thirty years ago, attitudes toward breast-feeding were far more relaxed. We were not expected to nurse on the first day. On the second day, we put our infants to our breasts for a few minutes every four hours so that our babies could suck if they wanted to. We knew that our babies would consume some colostrum, but we had no expectation that breast milk would be flowing. At the Beth Israel Hospital in Boston, an aide, Rose Finkelstein, brought my daughter to me for the first nursing session and was very supportive and encouraging. After several days, my milk was flowing, and Marissa began to gain weight.

In retrospect, my C-section provided an advantage to me in addition to the delivery of a healthy baby. That advantage was rest and relaxation time. Before childbirth, I was in graduate school full-time, I never napped, and I always filled any free time with projects or household tasks. I had planned to start a new semester full-time within a few weeks after delivery and had absolutely no plan to cut back on any part of my busy life.

But major surgery slowed me down. I stayed in the hospital for one week and got plenty of naps and rest while others changed diapers, washed baby clothes, and bathed my baby daughter. On the first day, I didn't nurse at all; I only held and cuddled her. For the next few days after that, I nursed her in short bouts every several hours. I was not laundering clothes, grocery shopping, or cooking. I was napping, reading, and watching TV. Friends and family visited, but I didn't have to make a pot of coffee or offer them cookies. On discharge, I was advised to stay close to home and to rest and recuperate as much as possible; driving was not recommended.

I had to become more realistic about my activity level. Instead of rushing back to a full-time school schedule, I cut back to half-time. Projects and household tasks took a backseat as I recuperated. I rested and napped to catch up on the sleep I was losing while nursing a baby in the middle of the night. I did not understand then that such recuperation and rest aided not only the healing process but also breast-feeding. Apparently, relaxation is a key ingredient for successful breast-feeding. Since I could do nothing to change my situation, I didn't stress about my lack of activity. I am convinced that breast-feeding was easy for me because I rested (albeit unintentionally), was relaxed as a result, and gave nursing the time it required.

Return to Yesteryear: Longer Hospital Stays?

I do not advocate longer hospital stays. But I will never try to convince a new mother that she is failing at breast-feeding when her milk is not flowing on day one, two, or three. I won't make a mother feel she is failing in nursing on day two as a reason to provide supplemental feedings or breast pumps. Breast-feeding is a natural function. It is driven by physiologic forces and not by economic forces. The pressures of medical economics have gone too far when new mothers are sad and frustrated in the first days of a newborn's life.

Babies Come without Agendas: Trust Your baby

Some things have not changed in ten thousand years, and you can easily put the process of breast-feeding a newborn baby on the top of that list. The one individual on the planet you can most trust about breast-feeding is not me, not the clinical practice guidelines in the hospital, not the lactation consultant. The one individual you can trust is your newborn baby. Luckily, the baby does not know that he has been born in the twenty-first century. The baby does not know about the economic, legal, and societal pressures. If your baby is content to sleep and pee off 10 percent of his birth weight over the first three to seven days, I would trust that baby. Any baby who is becoming dehydrated will not sleep contentedly; rather, the baby will let you know that he is having trouble. The baby's heart rate and respiratory rate will increase, and he will look weak and lack muscle tone. A baby content to lie and sleep and breathe quietly and maintain its muscle tone is saying, "I am quite all right."

Nursing is an Art, Not a Science

If nursing is as hard as we make it seem, we should all be amazed at how our species has managed to survive so well and how so many young mothers around the planet Earth are able to perform this task without pumps, supplements, doctors, and consultants. A newborn infant does not need any special input to tell it to breathe, urinate, defecate, or begin to suck. A new mother does not need any special input to figure out how to nurse. Like breathing, peeing, and pooping, breast-feeding is a basic biological act that would happen whether you delivered a baby on an isolated island with no assistance or in a modern hospital's maternity unit. The instruction manual for breast-feeding is already imprinted in your mind today as it was ten thousand years ago. Don't be afraid to trust yourself and your baby; both of you can be successful at breast-feeding if nature is allowed to take its course.

What are some steps you can take to ensure successful breast-feeding?

- For the first few weeks after your baby is born, sleep when the baby is sleeping. Just like ten thousand years ago, your body needs to recover from the birthing process, and resting your body will help you feel more relaxed when nursing.
- Drink plenty of water. Your body needs fluids to assist in the milk-making process. Water is your best bet.
- Begin nursing slowly. Breast-feeding is a slow process now just as it has been for eons. You do not want sore nipples on day four when your milk comes in.
- Avoid the stress of quickly resuming your active, busy life since stress is the most common factor that adversely affects successful nursing.
- Be encouraged by the thought that every member of your family, for thousands of years, has breast-fed their newborns successfully, or you would not be here today.

Parent Linda Y. wrote,

> *I remember Dr. Dan laughing when he told us that he asked Mike's cousin, Sam, what his baby brother ate and Sam answered, "I'm not sure, but it is something in my mother's armpit."*

Parent Courtney H. wrote,

> *Dr. Heller told me a story that first day in the hospital—about how children had been birthed since cavemen times and how the mother after giving birth would drag her bloody body down to the river to clean herself and it was because of this type of conditioning—neither the baby nor the mother had the need to feed in the first hours after birth—for me not to worry if my newborn didn't eat right away. That my body and my baby's body knew*

more than I did, that we had one expert in the room (he pointed to my baby) and that I was therefore NOT TO WORRY.

Parent Christine H. wrote:

When it came to breast feeding, Dr. Heller showed us what the doctors told his wife about when to breastfeed every time she had a child. Each time they told her something different.

Dr. Heller told us to feed the baby when he is hungry. The baby knows when he is hungry. And if we think the baby is so dumb that he does not know when he is hungry, it is better that we find that out now before we try to get him into Harvard.

6

Homeward Bound

Before a baby is born, her parents were well-defined, independent individuals. After her birth, parents return home as two very different people. Lao-tzu said, "When you stop being what you are, you become what you might be." This certainly applies to those who are delivering babies. They are becoming parents, a new, exciting but challenging role. Once at home from the hospital, the realization suddenly hits you that now you have new responsibilities. Nurses, doctors, or lactation personnel aren't in your home to give advice about the next steps.

Most parents probably think, "What do I know about parenting?" The answer is that we who become parents probably know much more than we think. With the knowledge that we have been on this planet for ten thousand years, it seems likely that most parenting skills are intuitive. Those skills are certainly intuitive for mammals like elephants and giraffes, who never shop in bookstores seeking the latest treatise on how to care for their young. And yet parents of human newborns usually have many questions and concerns. Obviously, we think at a much more sophisticated level than other mammals, but I believe that this current feeling that we need help is in part the result of the dispersion of the extended family.

Where Have All the Families Gone

For thousands of years, family units stayed together in regard to both their emotional ties as well as their physical proximity. Grandparents, aunts, uncles, and cousins were all together in the same group or village, and parenting skills were learned by observing others over a lifetime. Even last century, my parents lived in proximity to their parents, aunts, and uncles in Brooklyn. In the Bronx, my dad's sister raised her children with her in-laws in the same apartment. Actual physical and emotional supports were as far away as the next room.

Today, while the emotional connections continue, the geographic ones do not. In many cases, grandparents, aunts, and uncles are no longer close enough to hold the baby and give a physical helping hand. When we had our first child, my parents were in Florida, and Nancy's mother was in Texas; and between us, we have siblings and cousins in New York, southern California, New Jersey, Florida, Vermont, and Minnesota. We were in Boston, and although we were well educated, we had not spent much time around infants and children nor had we observed their growth and development.

To fill this presumed parenting knowledge gap, new parents read, talk to grandparents and friends, and listen to pediatricians and pediatric nurse-practitioners. Basically, new parents try to educate themselves using the resources at hand. Unfortunately, many times the advice you get may be contradictory, and confusion may reign.

Good News: It's Hard to Do Anything Wrong When There Is No Right

New parents ask, "What is the right way to care for a newborn baby?" The answer is simple: no "right" way exists. Cultural, social, and religious preferences may play a role in the advice one is given. I have the advantage of being a bit older. I have seen several waves of the "latest and most up-to-date parenting advice" go by, only to be renounced and ridiculed a few years later as old-school ideas and replaced by a new fad. Rather than becoming confused by all this inconstant advice, you should feel liberated and relaxed. Clearly, almost anything you do will have an advocate in the pediatric or lay press. Let's review some commonly asked questions in regard to newborn care. Are the answers difficult to discern? No. Give it a try, and more often than not, your answer won't be wrong. The key is to remember: for every parenting advice book on the bookstore shelf, there is another book which offers very different or even opposite advice. Since that is the case, parents clearly have wide latitude in selecting those techniques that are most comfortable for them.

All about Innies and Outies

For the last twenty-five years, the advice in the United States about caring for the umbilical stump was very clear and based on two rules. The first rule was to keep the umbilical cord dry until the cord fell off. The second rule was to apply alcohol twice daily around the umbilical stump to prevent infection. The first rule is inherently contradictory since a baby naturally urinates all over the cord (especially boys), thereby wetting it off and on throughout the day. Obviously, a parent can't instruct a newborn to keep his own cord dry. If a baby can pee on his cord, why can't we wet it by bathing? The answer is clear: the cord can and does get wet. As for the need to use alcohol, I wonder where our cave ancestors found alcohol to wipe on the cord. For that matter, why do we pay any attention to the cord at all? What did we do before alcohol?

Cord Care: Much Ado about Nothing

What is the origin of rules about cord care? Certainly, dogs, cats, elephants, or tigers do not shop in local pharmacies for rubbing alcohol to put on their newborns' cords. People around the world are fascinated by our umbilical cords. Different cultures treat cords in different ways. In Japan, parents are advised to put yellow baking flour on the cord. In Brazil, the recommended product is dried tobacco leaves. In India, powdered cow dung is the material of choice. Are these remedies necessary? The simple answer is a definite <u>no</u>. Throughout the mammalian species, the cord dries up on its own and falls off without any special encouragement from us.

So why did cord care ever become an issue? Occasionally, the cord may become infected superficially and have a fetid odor. Reasonable cleanliness and washing will usually clear this up. Do not be afraid to move the cord side to side when washing. Debris collects under the cord, and that debris can become malodorous around the umbilical stump. Simple washing with or without alcohol is the solution.

Commonly, some bleeding may occur as the cord separates over the first or second week of life, and that bleeding looks like dried blood inside baby's diaper. On occasion, a slow dripping of blood happens. Applying mild pressure with a cotton ball will stop this bleeding just as light pressure stops bleeding from a razor nick or a scratch. In the event that the bleeding does not stop, a visit to your pediatrician for cauterization of the cord is warranted. Cauterization is the use of a chemical or electrical agent that will burn the end of the bleeding vessel. This technique does not cause pain for a baby because the cord tissue has no nerve fibers.

Of much greater concern is the rare incidence of a deep infection of the cord. Bacteria have the potential to enter the umbilical artery or umbilical vein, whose cut ends are in the stump. Such infection can travel up these vessels and into the infant's body. This unusual infection usually happens as a complication after a catheter has been inserted into the umbilical artery. Catheter placement in the umbilical artery is a procedure performed on ill newborns in a neonatal intensive care unit. An infection of this sort is associated with fever, local redness, swelling, and, possibly, pus draining from the umbilical stump. Such symptoms mandate a call to your pediatric provider, who will usually advise a trip to an emergency room.

A final problem is the cord that decides it simply won't fall off and go away. If at two weeks of age the cord is not drying up at all, your provider may cauterize the cord to ensure that the drying up process comes to completion. Rarely, the cord may take several weeks to finally separate, but this delay causes no adverse consequences. Except for the situations noted above, the truth is that the cord does not require any special treatment, and it will fall off naturally whether parents use cow dung or alcohol.

A Few Tips (Pun Intended) about Circumcision

This topic raises (pun intended) more social, cultural, religious, and psychological questions than most issues of newborn care. The obvious answer is that circumcision is not necessary. We know this for two reasons. No other mammals circumcise their young, and more importantly, insurance companies consider it cosmetic surgery and will not cover the cost of the procedure. In fact, the only "medical" advice that everyone agrees on is <u>not</u> to circumcise an infant with certain abnormalities of the head or shaft of the penis. Some boys are born with an abnormal exit of the urethra. In this situation, the urethra does not exit at the tip of the penis, but exits on the underside of the shaft. To repair this anomaly, surgeons can use the foreskin tissue as a flap to cover and reconstruct the defect. This type of abnormality is a significant medical problem and not merely cosmetic; even insurance companies will pay for the procedure to repair penile abnormalities.

At the other end of the circumcision issue, from a medical viewpoint, is the older child with a very tight foreskin and as a result, painful swelling of the head of the penis called a phimosis. In this situation, the "medical" advice is yes, that child should be circumcised.

That is the end of the medical input on this topic but by no means the end of the discussion.

So where did this circumcision idea come from? A religious friend of mine tells me that in Eden, Adam did not have a foreskin covering the tip of his penis. When he "sinned," he broke his covenant with God and was expelled from paradise. As he left, he covered his penis with a fig leaf to show his shame. Thereafter, every man was born with a fig leaf (substituted with the foreskin) covering his penis. Much later, God tells Abraham that in order to reestablish his covenant with God, Abraham must cut off the foreskin. By removing the foreskin, each individual is accepting a covenant with God that was lost when Adam sinned. Just as an aside, Abraham apparently was forty years old at the time and performed the surgery on himself with a sharpened stone. Ouch! I am sure there are many other stories and different references in different cultures. But the truth is there is no medical reason for newborn circumcisions.

Getting Back to the Point (Pun Intended)

Knowing the truth, however, does not always help us make a decision. As I said, social, cultural, religious, and psychiatric viewpoints are more determinative of the process. For me, the most compelling argument I have heard over the years is "Like father, like son." It is probably more important for a child to look like his dad than like the other kids in the neighborhood. If the father is circumcised, it probably makes sense for the son to be circumcised as well; and if the father is uncircumcised, then it probably makes sense for the son to be uncircumcised as well.

Once the decision to circumcise has been made, parents are confronted with more decision making. "Do we need anesthesia? And if so, should we use a topical pain reducing cream, or should we inject anesthetic at the base of the penis to block all nerve transmission of pain? Or maybe we will be fine with just a little alcohol for the baby to suck on."

The latter approach saves the possible complications of injections, such as a hematoma at the penile base (ouch). My personal preference is not to make a medically unnecessary procedure more complicated with injections of anesthetics or other invasive procedures. The issue is clearly related to our individual perceptions about pain. Which is worse: a needle piercing the skin and the injection of an anesthetic that initially swells the soft tissue space at the base of the penis, or the quick performance of the procedure? Obviously, that choice is all in our minds as individuals. Some of us prefer Novocain at the dentist, and some of us do not. In the end, much as the parents are asked to make an informed choice on this matter, it probably makes the most sense to ask the surgeon, doctor, or moyel, "How are you most comfortable performing the procedure?" I would trust the judgment of the person who will perform the circumcision.

Straight Talk (Pun Intended) about Circumcision Care

Caring for a newly circumcised infant is simple. While parents are frequently given an instruction sheet that is two to three pages long, one really does not need anything but a little Vaseline. The tip of the penis will look bright red and inflamed initially; over the following days, the circumcision site will develop a yellow crust. This crust eventually comes off, and after two weeks, the penis is beautiful. Despite the fact that this raw tissue sits in a diaper with urine and stool, I have never seen a circumcision become infected. The only common problem I have seen after circumcision is the development of a penile adhesion. Weeks and months after the actual procedure, the skin along the shaft of the penis may adhere, as part of the healing process, to the tip of the penis. Your pediatrician can ease this adhesion apart and then apply Vaseline to lessen the likelihood of a recurrence.

Over the River and through the Woods: When Can I Take My Baby Outdoors?

Like so many newborn care questions, the answer to the question of when to take your baby outside varies depending to whom the question is addressed. At discharge, some hospitals instruct a new mother to keep her baby indoors for anywhere from two to six weeks. That is an isolating and depressing way to begin life as a new parent. Others advise outdoor time as long as the baby is not "in a crowd." Rarely is a crowd defined. Classically, three's a crowd, once again limiting the ability to go out and socialize.

Clearly, if this is the third or fourth child in a family, she is immediately in a crowd of other children merely by being at home. And if this child is born in a third or fourth world village, she is probably outdoors from the beginning and living amidst crowds of people.

Mothers with older children do not suddenly tell them that everyone has to stay in the house for any length of time. Three-year-olds are not told to find their own way back and forth from play groups and daycare programs because their mothers have to stay indoors with their new baby siblings. The obvious conclusion is that a newborn can be taken outdoors immediately.

In fact, new mothers benefit from being outside, breathing some fresh air and socializing. Being forced to remain isolated and stay inside can worsen postpartum depression. It is a disservice to a mom's mental health to have a rule forbidding her from getting fresh air for her baby.

What Temperature Should I Keep the House, and How Should I Dress the Baby? Presumably, you intend for this newborn baby to remain your child for a lifetime and live with you for quite a number of years. The truth is you should keep your house temperature the same as before and make no special adjustments for the infant. Children grow up in igloos in Alaska and in thatch homes in South Africa. Our species has been able to adjust in every part of the planet, and our newborns follow suit.

In regard to how to dress a baby, I believe it was Dr. Spock who suggested that one should dress the baby as one thinks one should and then remove one layer. Most parents tend to overdress their infants. Babies are a metabolic ball of fire. During the first months of her life, a baby is growing at a faster rate than she will ever do again. One of the reasons a baby feeds every three hours is that the rapidity of her early growth requires a frequent refueling of her system. Just as a coal locomotive steaming down the tracks needs a coalman to keep throwing more fuel in the engine, so too does a newborn speed full steam ahead 24/7. The result of this metabolic action is the generation of heat. Babies have a higher basal body temperature than adults. Overdressing newborns can make it difficult to dissipate this heat. You and I sweat to get rid of our excess heat, but babies don't sweat in the same way. A lot of heat is dissipated through the scalp, and at times, a baby's head and hair are wet. Therefore, do not overdress babies.

General Maintenance of a Newborn: How to Keep That "Like New" Look

No new parent is home from the hospital for very long before the newborn becomes covered with pee, poop, and refluxed feedings. She will also get a snotty nose and goopy pus-filled eyes. Add sucking blisters on her lips, a red buttocks, and raw cheeks. By week's end, that beautiful baby is not so beautiful. Some routine maintenance is necessary to restore that lovely new baby look. Many nonperfumed moisturizing creams are safe to use on a baby's skin. Excessive bathing can dry out the skin and is not necessary. Thicker creams are available for the baby's buttocks to protect it from the irritation of multiple loose stools. Keep in mind that every rash does not need a treatment and sucking blisters are normal and will resolve on their own.

Mission Control—All Systems are GO (Pun Intended)!

Peeing and pooping are first on the agenda of daily maintenance. Your newborn will quite quickly be "going" at either end fairly frequently. All systems are definitely go, and that is a good sign.

My Baby Seems Pissed Off

In regard to urine, you can expect wet diapers every three hours. In fact, urination is the reason for changing diapers frequently. The brand of the diaper does not matter. For practical reasons, most parents choose disposable diapers instead of reusable cloth diapers. The only problem with the absorbent materials in disposable diapers is that the chemical absorbents can make crystal-like particles congeal on the surface. All too many times, I have taken a late-night call saying that "My baby is peeing crystals." The answer is that the baby is peeing normally, and the diaper is making the crystals. No human baby has ever peed out a crystal so big it is visible to the naked eye.

The color is sometimes a concern for parents, especially when they observe an orange-red color in the diaper and worry that their baby is bleeding. Actually, babies excrete a large amount of phosphates in their urine. The reason for the high concentration of phosphates is that both breast milk and formula, a baby's only food, contain a lot of calcium in the form of calcium-phosphate salts. Unutilized minerals are excreted in stool and urine. When these excreted phosphate salts in the urine are exposed to air, the urine turns orangey red. When adults and children pee in a toilet, the urine color is diluted, and our urine is not exposed to air for very long. However, when these phosphate salts are sitting in a diaper and exposed to air, they become orange-red and are mistaken for blood in the urine.

Blood actually looks like blood in most cases. Sometimes, in the diaper of a baby girl, parents will observe blood that comes from their baby's vagina. Baby girls have full-fledged levels of female hormones at birth that rapidly decline over the first week. At times, the fall in hormone levels leads to withdrawal bleeding from the baby's uterus, just as what happens when one is cycling on birth control pills. The blood is usually mixed with mucus and the bleeding does not last very long. If uncertain about the blood and its source, you should call your pediatrician.

What's the Scoop about Poop?

Baby poop may surprise new parents. Breast-fed babies may poop eight times in one day, usually in the middle of a feeding. On the other hand, they may poop just once in an eight-day period. I answer more questions from new and old parents about poop than any other single issue. Parents are concerned about the color, the texture, the frequency, the odor, and the consistency of this excretory product. Where did our fascination for this end product come from?

I tell my patients an apocryphal story. When God handed Moses the Eleven Commandments, number eleven was "Thou shalt poop every day on a regular basis and make your parents proud." When Moses returned after destroying the original tablets, he asked God whether they could eliminate this eleventh commandment. God replied, "As long as poops are soft, I guess I don't care how often you have them." That is the reason we only have Ten Commandments.

Truthfully, poops of breast-fed babies are likely to be runny and out of the diaper in an instant because they are so watery. Be prepared to change a diaper as well as the socks of a newborn after a normal stool. On rare occasions, the stool may have some blood. In most instances, this blood is due to local irritation or a rectal fissure and is of no great consequence, but you should call your pediatrician to discuss the situation if you see blood.

In bottle-fed babies, especially those on soy formulas, the stool may become excessively hard. Hard stools can be uncomfortable for a baby to pass, and the passing may cause a rectal fissure or tear. If this occurs, a tablespoon of Karo syrup added to the formula twice a day may provide a sufficient softening effect by pulling more moisture into the stool. In general, I do not recommend soy formulas because of the issue of constipation.

A Clean Sweep

Parents frequently ask about the best method to wash pee or poop from their baby's bottom and what to put on that bottom after cleaning. If there is a real mess, nothing beats a quick trip to the sink or a rapid tub bath to wash off the infant's bottom. For a less messy bum, wipe the infant's buttocks with either a wet cloth or a non-perfumed wipe. Just using some baby oil on a cotton ball is a great way to wipe off the baby's soiled skin without abrading or irritating the surface. The cotton ball and oil actually lubricate the skin and clean the baby at the same time. After cleaning, smear on a layer of protective emollient. Whether one uses Vaseline, Desitin, Balmex, or some other brand makes little difference.

Some people prefer to protect these areas with powder. Corn starch and talc are frequently used. The problem with powders is that babies may inhale the particulate matter of the powder as one shakes the powder to apply it. If you prefer powder, it is better to pour it out and pick up a "pinch of powder" at a time and rub it in where necessary.

Rub-a-dub-dub

Parents also often ask about how often to bathe their babies. Bathing actually removes natural oils from one's skin; medically, we advise parents whose child might have eczema to bathe less often. But obviously, all babies need to be bathed, especially when covered with poop from head to toe. Sometimes, parents find themselves bathing their babies two or more times in one day. For instance, you bathe your baby because she is covered with poop; immediately after the bath, she needs to be fed again. That feeding stimulates her gastrocolic reflex, and she becomes soiled all over again. In this situation, the advice is to bathe your baby every several minutes! After this, she may not poop again for a few days, which is perfectly normal, and she would not need a bath for at least two days. Most definitely, there is no rule about how often to bathe your baby. Use common sense and your senses of sight and smell.

Goopy Eyes and Runny Noses—Welcome to the World of Babies!

Babies have small nasal passages and small lacrimal ducts that drain fluid and mucus from the nose and eyes. Because those passages and ducts are small, they are sometimes overwhelmed by secretions, and the result is noisy breathing and nasal discharge or accumulation of pus in the eyes and nose. More often than not, these are superficial infections that require no treatment.

At birth, the babies' eyes are treated with antibiotic ointment to protect the eyes from any infection acquired as the babies moved through the vaginal canal. If a baby's eyes become pussy in the first two weeks, the most reasonable step is to wipe away the pus rather than to re-treat the eyes. Your pediatrician will reassess the situation and re-treat if necessary when you bring your baby for the two-week visit.

Runny noses occur with such frequency that we should probably label them as normal. A baby's nose is in the forefront of her immune system. Her nose is the first to encounter all types of particulate matter and foreign bodies and responds by making mucus and secretions. Babies always seem to have congested noses. Unfortunately, hospital nurseries give parents a cute blue rubber aspirator to suck out this mucus. That aspirator only irritates the nasal membranes, and the irritation causes the production of more and more mucus. Save the aspirator as a bathtub toy. If a baby's congestion is very noisy, use a few drops of salt water, which will soften dried mucus and cause the baby to sneeze the mucus up and out. Parents are usually astonished by the quantity of mucus that one or two sneezes can generate. Saltwater nose drops are easily and most economically made by mixing a teaspoon of salt in an eight-ounce glass of water. Naturally, saltwater nose drops are also available commercially in pharmacies. In any event, the noisy congestion sounds probably bother the parents more than they bother the baby.

Safety First

I have three tips about safety. First, buy or borrow a proper baby car seat for your car, and *use it*. Make this purchase before the mother and the baby leave the hospital or birthing center. The American Academy of Pediatrics website, www.AAP.org, has terrific information on the proper baby car seat for your vehicle and the proper installation.

Second, make an emergency or fire evacuation plan with other adult household members. Who will go for the baby? Where will you meet? How can you exit if the usual egress is blocked? Is there a safe way to throw your infant out of a window to the other parent or another adult? These plans should be in place before the unlikely event of an emergency like a fire. Unfortunately, tragedies do occur, and the best plan is to be prepared. Your local firehouse will be interested to know you have a baby in your home or apartment and may give you a "Tot Finder" sticker to put in the window of the baby's room.

Third, carry your baby as if she is a football. Tuck her feet under your arm and cradle her head in your hand. In this way, her head is in the midline of your body, and your fingers are in front. The reason for this portage position is this: since you will be tired and up at least a few times during the night, you want to protect your baby's head from being the first object to bump against a wall or door frame.

Now at home with your new joy and pride
You do <u>not</u> have a new owner's guide
Wiping pee, poop, and snot
Complex it is not
Trust your feelings, it's all there inside.

Parent Judith S. wrote,

> *I gave birth in a birthing center and needed to schedule an appointment with our pediatrician within 48 hours because of early discharge from the birthing center. The purpose was to receive a shot and a newborn checkup and to remove the umbilical cord clamp. Unfortunately, although Dr. Heller was in the office that day, we couldn't fit into his schedule and so had the visit with another doctor in the practice. She was nice and competent but told us to our great disappointment that we would have to go back to Cambridge Hospital to have the cord clamp removed because a "special tool" was required that had to match the type of cord clamp our daughter had, and this special tool was not available at Centre Pediatrics.*

> *Well, just about then, Dr. Dan peeped in the door to meet the newest member of the family and he greeted her with irrepressible joy. "Who does your hair?" he asks this two-day-old with abundant spiked hair.*

> *When appraised of our current cord clamp dilemma, he immediately waved his hand in the air. "I have that tool." Once again, we were saved by the man with all the answers! He disappeared and quickly reappeared with the tool: a Leatherman—and quite matter of factly, he proceeded to pry off the umbilical cord clamp while my tiny daughter looked placidly on. It was a moment of Heller magic—so simple, so basic, so beautiful.*

Parent Linda Y. wrote,

> *When we told Dr. Dan that more than a few Brookline ladies had reprimanded us for taking our baby out in the cold, Dr. Dan simply told us to tell those ladies that people have babies in Alaska!*

Parent Lisa L. wrote,

> *I remember sitting at the orientation for parents-to-be … a room full of highly hormonal, pregnant women, holding their bellies, firing questions at Dr. Dan. One woman asks…. "There are different mattresses for the crib, some are firmer than others, what is the best degree of firmness for the baby?"*

Just as I thought ... "Oh no, I hadn't thought of this! What if I got the wrong one? Will they take it back? I'll have to just buy a second one!"..... Dr. Dan said, "Get the one that feels most like the ground, because most babies in the world sleep on the ground."

At that moment, I know he was the guy for me. I breathed a huge sigh of relief, and knew that I could do this mom thing, and I could do it well.

7

Day Three

Prepare to Outsource Food and Acquire Liquid: Check Brain, Kidneys, Adrenals, Pancreas, Liver, and Intestines

The third day of life represents an entirely new and different set of circumstances for both the baby and the mother. On the first day, Mother Nature issued a free pass regarding the fluid needs of the infant. The first baby breaths pushed fluid from the lungs into the baby's body; the infant is filled with enough fluid to allow him to rest and recuperate from his efforts to undergo transition to life on earth. Slowly, over the first three days, he has been peeing off that extra fluid. Typically, between days three and four, he will begin to need sustenance. The timing of a baby's need for sustenance varies considerably. While many babies show interest in nursing after three or four days because they have urinated off their fluid overload, some babies are still content to sleep and recuperate for as long as seven days; those babies have not yet rid themselves of their extra fluid and continue to have frequent wet diapers.

In the first ten minutes of life, the respiratory and cardiovascular systems begin to function. Now on day three (or later, depending on the baby), the gastrointestinal system has to be tested.

The gastrointestinal system may seem rather simple at first glance. Every human has two body openings connected to the gastrointestinal system: one at the top end called the mouth and a second opening at the bottom end called the rectum. What goes in must come out, and in between, some calories are absorbed for growth and energy. What a gross oversimplification! In actuality, the gastrointestinal system stretches almost from head to toe and not just from mouth to rectum.

I'm Hungry; I'm Thirsty

In the human brain, in an area called the hypothalamus, are cells that are specialized to sense and react to hunger and other cells that are specialized to sense and react to thirst. These cells in the hypothalamus respond to information from a myriad of sources. When blood sugar levels rise and fall, hormones are released or withdrawn and influence the hypothalamus. Hunger cells receive information from several sources including fat cells, blood sugar level, endocrine glands (like the thyroid), and distention level of the stomach and bowel. These sources advise hunger cells whether the body is running on empty or feeling quite full and satiated. The thyroid gland in the neck sets the overall rate of metabolism for the body, and the level of thyroid gland activity affects the workings of the hypothalamus. In like manner, the central nervous system will signal a feeling of hunger or fullness depending on the degree of distention of the wall of the stomach.

The kidneys monitor fluid volume in the body and, together with hormones from the adrenal gland, affect changes that make you feel thirsty. The blood pressure in the carotid artery that brings blood to the brain has pressure sensors to also advise the organism about the fluid volume status.

When we feel hungry, thirsty, satisfied, or sated, that feeling is the result of a number of physiologic processes. The need for fluid and the need for calories are adjusted by positive and negative feedback systems that work from minute to minute. Most of the fine-tuning of these processes occurs at the level of the cells or the organs involved. For example, if our kidneys are receiving a large blood flow, they react by excreting fluid as urine. If, on the other hand, the blood flow is low, our kidneys react by reabsorbing fluid. Depending on whether the muscular wall of the stomach is stretched or relaxed affects whether we are hungry or not. Again, this information is sent to the brain, which converts this information into a feeling of hunger or satiety.

You can be sure that this is a simplification of a very complex process. Medical schools would have been easy if I only had to know this much. The point is that the feeling of hunger or thirst involves a complex interaction of many organs and monitoring structures that exist throughout the body and report to the commander-in-chief, the brain. The brain reacts to information and signals from many sources; and for the first three days of a baby's life, the signals to a baby's brain will indicate that the fluid and caloric needs are being fully met, and all is well. Depending on the information that is received, messages are sent out by nerves from the brain to the mouth, and a baby's reaction is to begin to suck or eat.

Word from the Front Lines: We Need Reinforcements

On his third day of life, signals from a baby's body organs and sensors begin to change. His fluid volume is beginning to fall, and calories are not as readily available as his fat stores are diminished. At birth, the baby has extra fluid as well as extra fat. The fluid is stored both in the cells and vascular system, and the fat has been stored throughout the body. The extra fluid has ensured that the vascular system is intact, and the extra fat has provided a reserve of calories. These reserves of fluid and fat are used during the first days of life and are slowly diminishing and, eventually, like all reserves, will run out.

The time has come for the infant to turn his attention to revving up the gastrointestinal system. As with many other acquired skills, this requires the successful coordination of many parts. His mouth has to learn how to open and latch on to his mother's nipple; at the same time, he has to figure out how to swallow and move the colostrum and breast milk down the esophagus into his stomach. His stomach has to learn to close off its far end; milk needs to remain in his stomach for a while so that it can be curdled by acids and then mixed and digested into a slush that can be squeezed into the intestines.

The complexity of this task is increased as the baby's pancreas has to squirt in some amylase to digest starches, and his liver has to add a bit of bile. Next, his intestines have to begin to absorb his broken down fat, protein, and carbohydrate complexes, transfer them to his circulation, and deliver them to his liver and tissues. His tissues choose whether to utilize these nutrients or to store them for future use. Residual, unused particulate matter has to be moved down his bowel to be deposited in his diaper at a later date.

Finally, the mission is accomplished, but the entire cycle begins again in three to four hours. As with many newly acquired natural processes, coordinating all these systems takes some time. What may appear to be eat, drink, pee, and poop actually represents an amazing coordinated effort of the neurologic, endocrine, muscular, renal, and endocrine systems. Not surprisingly, this whole process takes a few days to begin to work efficiently. Also, remember that what has been mentioned above represents only half the challenge. While these systems are beginning to mature and operate in the baby, new systems are also becoming operative in the mother.

Let's See What These Breasts Can Do

At the beginning of adolescence, females notice the development of breasts. Those breasts require girls and women to modify their clothing and make other accommodations in their lifestyles regarding sports and work. Women carry their breasts around for seventy years or more; however, on the third or fourth day of a baby's life, breasts have their really big day and declare their usefulness. Despite all the jokes and what anyone else might tell you, nature has given women breasts for one primary reason and that is to provide nutrition and fluid to babies. That might sound very simple and straightforward, but the breast-feeding system, like the infant's gastrointestinal system, is quite complex. Also, like a newborn's gastrointestinal system, a new mom's breasts have not been tested despite their age.

Breast milk does not just suddenly appear out of the blue. During pregnancy, hormonal changes occur that lead to the maturation of the milk-producing glands in the breast. Women notice that their breasts enlarge and feel different as pregnancy progresses. The breasts are being made ready for the task of nursing. However, at the moment of birth, a woman's body is filled with hormones from the placenta that actually block the ability to make milk. Over the first three to four days of a baby's life, mom's kidneys urinate these blocking hormones out of mom's system. At this point, cells in mom's brain begin to produce and release lactating hormones that travel via arteries to the breasts. Lactating hormones stimulate the glandular tissue of the breasts to begin the production of milk. The system, however, is more complex than that.

Just as the feedback systems in a baby's gastrointestinal system involve nerves and endocrine organs, so too is the making of milk influenced by other factors. Mom's fluid status is monitored by volume and pressure receptors just like her baby's fluid status. If mom has inadequate fluid, she will not make adequate milk. If mom is overtired, milk may be delayed. If mom is overly stressed, milk production may be less than expected. I will never forget when Matthew was about six weeks old. Nancy was nursing him for about ten minutes. I reminded her that she should finish up since we had planned to shop for a new mattress. She looked at me and said, "I haven't let down yet." I had no idea what she was talking about. She explained to me that sometimes, even though Matthew is sucking away like crazy, she is somehow holding back and not letting the milk flow out. Other times, the milk would be squirting out of her breasts and into his face before he could latch on. I realized then that there is a lot that goes on between the brain and the breast that we do not control and do not know how to measure.

It's easy to say "just relax." However, as with so many situations, it is not so easy to "just relax."

Take-home Lessons on Relaxation from Cardiac Rehab

In 1990, I had the "good fortune" to have a heart attack. Although I hadn't always taken good care of my body, at that time I was jogging four days a week, maintaining an appropriate weight, and not smoking. But I was stressed because of my father's recent illness and death and my senior partner's retirement from our pediatric practice.

Good Fortune from Bad Problems

An important part of the treatment following my heart attack was a cardiac rehabilitation program. That program included visits from a nutritionist for dietary advice, an exercise program to get in shape, and a psychiatric program to learn about stress reduction. The "good fortune" for me was learning that stress was a major contributing factor to my heart attack and learning how to manage the stresses of life.

Avoid, Alter, or Accept

One of the easiest concepts of stress reduction is the realization that only three solutions exist for any problem that creates stress: avoid, alter, or accept. Let's say someone has to catch a flight, and time is getting short. He drives to the airport but is delayed by a red traffic light. Ready to push the pedal to the metal, he looks at his watch. He is agitated and stressed. Is this moment of stress necessary? He has no options. The light is red, and he cannot change that. In this situation, the only option is to sit at the wheel and accept the fact of a few minutes' delay. However, if he sees the light turn red up ahead and knows of an alternative right turn before that light, he can take that turn. In that way, he is altering the situation, and this is the less stressful alternative. Finally, he could have taken a taxi to the airport and avoided the stress of driving his own car.

For almost every crisis that occurs in life, to avoid, to alter, and to accept are the options, and one should not take long to come to a choice.

These concepts are applicable to almost every child behavior and parenting issue that will develop as you raise your child. Take breast-feeding as an example. If you want to breast-feed, understand and accept that you can succeed just as billions and billions of women before you have succeeded. Do not focus on exactly when your milk will come in or whether your baby will gain weight in a month; these are stressful thoughts that may interfere with your ultimate success because stress about breast-feeding or about other aspects of your life can interfere with your production of breast milk. Altering or avoiding the choice to breast-feed is also an option for the future; you can always switch to bottle-feeding. But if you elect to nurse, you can succeed just as well as if you elect to formula feed, especially if you don't allow stress to interfere.

Enjoy the Moment

The second lesson of stress reduction is to enjoy every moment. The cardiac rehab exercise program focused on yoga, tai chi, relaxation response, and tension-relaxation techniques. These exercises all began with taking several deep breaths and reminding yourself that you are alive and breathing. Breathing is the initial focus of each of these stress-reducing exercises. Surely, the premise is that if you are not breathing correctly, you have a much bigger problem than whatever problem you are facing at the moment. The second common denominator of all these is that they required going through movements, poses, thoughts, and transitions that have to be memorized When you are undergoing transition from the "cat stretch" to "cobra position," you must concentrate; you cannot think about problems at the office.

If you focus on what you are doing instead of what you are not doing, you will have less stress. Christie, my cardiac rehab nurse, told me, "You can meditate all day." I did not see how I could "meditate all day" and still be a successful pediatrician. Over time, I came to realize that if meditation means focus, then it does not matter what one focuses on. Whether the focus is to follow the many steps involved in tai chi or to listen and relate to a patient in the office, the result is the same: you are involved in the moment and not aggravated about things in the past or the future. The result is the reduction of stress and an enjoyable day full of accomplishments.

On the third day after giving birth, I meet so many moms who are either crying or on the brink of tears. They are openly stressed and unhappy. They were usually barraged for forty-eight hours with an enormous amount of advice about breast-feeding. Frequently, that advice puts an enormous amount of unnecessary pressure on you as a new mom to manufacture milk quickly. This heavy pressure from hospital staff to initiate the nursing process and to use breast pumps to make your milk come in sooner than nature intended induce stress but do not necessarily lead to faster milk production. Unfortunately, for many new moms, just the opposite transpires, and new mothers are less successful at nursing due to the stresses involved.

Day three will not be so stressful if days one and two are spent taking in fluids and resting and enjoying the moment. A mom's body is undergoing major changes to become "unpregnant," but this does not mean a mom's body will be as it was before pregnancy. After having the body of a gestating woman for nine months, every new mom is about to undergo transition into the body of a lactating woman. Just as the first change took her some time to become accustomed to, so will this second change.

I know you will nurse successfully. I know this because our species have nursed successfully for thousands of years. It will happen as naturally as your breathing.

What you must remember is that from day three to day six, both you and your baby are learning. Both you and your baby are undergoing transitions to a new physical state that you have never dealt with before. Like the first ten minutes of life, major changes are occurring, and major changes take some time. Trust that nature has provided that timeframe in which to accomplish this transition. Day three is just an early step on the long road of parenting. Take this step slowly and enjoy it.

- The transition to lactation begins, but don't expect your breasts to be overflowing at this point.

- All great journeys begin with a first step, and being home with your baby is step number one.

- I never breast-fed anyone, but Nancy did. Her advice is to "drink plenty of fluids and rest as much as you can."

- Let sleeping babies lay. You don't have to rush yourself or the baby to learn how to nurse before either of your bodies is ready.

- Breast-feeding is a learning process, and both the mother and the baby are new at it. Over the next few weeks, you will both become more adept.

8

First-Week Issues Out of Your Control

One of the most important lessons of parenting is that, as parents, we don't control many aspects of our children's lives. This becomes very apparent in the first week of an infant's life. For example, heart murmurs may occur or become apparent on day two or three, and jaundice many times does not occur until day three to seven. Common clinical issues that arise in the first week are blood sugar instability and inability to maintain body temperature. Of course, babies lose weight during this week despite your best efforts. A fever may develop, or an infant may have signs of an infection unrelated to anything her parents are doing.

But I am troubled because the blame for some of these problems is cast on the mother. I have heard medical professionals claim that jaundice, low blood sugar, and fever are all due to failure to make breast milk on day one and two. Such a claim is not accurate since no woman has milk on day one. Unfortunately, without a solid explanation for some of these clinical problems, these medical professionals and hospital defense systems turn to the mother as the likely cause, especially the nursing mother. However, mothers are innocent of these charges, and it is worth looking at the real causes to allay any guilt a new mother may feel.

Here Today, Gone Tomorrow, and Then Here Again the Next Day: Heart Murmurs

As mentioned earlier, the circulation of blood in the fetus is significantly different from that of a newborn. While in utero, the heart of the fetus is relieved of any responsibility to push blood through the lungs to oxygenate that blood. Instead, the flow of blood bypasses the fetal lungs by passing through a patent (open) blood vessel called the ductus arteriosus. On the first day of life, pediatricians commonly hear heart murmurs or extra sounds from the baby's heart. Murmurs usually occur when the flow of blood through the heart is either turbulent or traveling in an abnormal direction. Frequently, a murmur heard on the first day of life is due to a failure of the ductus arteriosus to close immediately after birth. The flow through this patent (open) vessel is turbulent and gives rise to a murmur. This type of murmur is usually gone by the second day of life. Often, a pediatrician will not even mention the presence of this murmur so as not to worry parents about a normal occurrence. At other times, the murmur may *not* sound like a simple ductus, and a further evaluation will be performed. Most of the time, no murmur is heard at all on the first day of life.

To a certain degree, what the heart sounds like on the second day of life is more important than what the heart sounds on the first. By the second day of life, innocent murmurs of the ductus arteriosus are usually gone, but new murmurs may become apparent. The murmurs discovered on day two or three of life are more commonly due to defects in the muscular wall of the heart that separates the right and left sides. These are called atrio-septal or ventriculo-septal defects. At this point, an in-depth analysis is generally performed to determine how significant the problem is.

As soon as a heart murmur is mentioned, most every member of the family becomes concerned and upset. The good news is that almost all heart defects discovered at this time either resolve over time or are amenable to surgical correction.

A Jaundiced View of the World

The single most common problem that develops after delivery is jaundice of the newborn.

Jaundice is characterized by the yellowing of the skin due to a buildup of a compound called bilirubin in the blood. During their first week, almost all babies develop some degree of jaundice that usually is of no consequence. However, if a baby's bilirubin reaches certain elevated levels, the bilirubin can cause permanent damage to the central nervous system. For this significant reason, we monitor newborns for their color.

If jaundice appears, all too often moms are told that their babies are not getting enough to eat and drink, and the implication is that the mothers are the cause of the jaundice. Moms are urged to nurse longer and offer supplemental feeds to get rid of the jaundice. In this situation, the blame is placed unfairly but squarely on the new moms. Basic information about the physiology of jaundice should convince every new mom who is reading this book that she is not guilty.

Every single day of every human's life, we make new red blood cells and break down old ones. Over a thirty-day period, we replace every red blood cell in our bodies. When a red blood cell is broken down, it releases a compound called bilirubin into the bloodstream. Bilirubin is picked up by the liver and converted by liver enzymes into a nontoxic product that is secreted into the intestines and removed as waste from the body in the stool. As long as one's liver is working normally, bilirubin does not build up in the blood, and one does not appear to have yellow skin.

Bilirubin is handled in a different manner by fetuses. A fetus also makes new red blood cells and destroys old ones, but while the fetus is in the uterus, it returns the released bilirubin to the mother through the placenta. The mother's liver then processes this bilirubin and converts it into waste. Thus, on the first day of life, babies appear perfectly clear of any jaundice. Jaundice levels rise in three- to seven-day-old newborns because the newborns' livers do not have the proper enzymes in place ready to perform during the first few days of life. In fact, the liver enzymes develop partly in response to the rise in bilirubin over the first few days. Essentially, a baby's liver is in an immature resting state since the maternal liver was processing the bilirubin for the fetus.

I view the problem of jaundice of the newborn as a race between the rate of generation of bilirubin in the baby versus the time it takes for the newborn's liver to gear up and make the enzymes necessary to detoxify the bilirubin. If the liver begins its work sooner, then the level of jaundice never reaches a significant level. If the liver is slow to activate its enzymes, jaundice may reach levels that need to be treated.

The bottom line is we are all waiting for the baby's liver to rev up and cope with one of its principal tasks. Why should anyone think that jaundice is a problem of inadequate fluid? Yes, the truth is that encouraging the gastrointestinal tract to work will stimulate the liver to process bilirubin. But it is equally true that new mothers have no milk during the first few days after childbirth. And it is frequently very difficult, if not impossible, to force a one- or two-day-old to suck down any fluid since the baby is over-hydrated, very sleepy, and disinterested in sucking.

Normally, the rise in bilirubin does not reach toxic levels before the infant's liver is capable of processing that bilirubin. However, sometimes, the bilirubin load is greater than normal due to physiologic factors out of anyone's control. If this rise in bilirubin occurs before the infant's liver has developed the ability to break down bilirubin, then jaundice becomes apparent and medical intervention becomes necessary. The major factor adding to bilirubin load is the blood group differences between the mother and the fetus (and birth induced cephalohematomas). At times, the blood group of the mother is different from that of the fetus. If intact, red blood cells from the fetus cross the placental barrier and enter the mother, then the maternal immune system may make an antibody to destroy that cell. These antibodies can cross over into the fetus and cause an increased rate of breakdown of red blood cells. This increase will lead to a more rapid rise of bilirubin than is generally expected, and significant jaundice may occur.

Another source for increased bilirubin load is a cephalohematoma. A cephalohematoma results from the fetal head being used as a ramrod against the cervix at delivery. A hematoma is an area of bleeding under the skin that collects in a closed space. A cephalohematoma is like a giant black-and-blue mark or a bruise. The blood cells in the hematoma break down and thereby add an extra load of bilirubin above and beyond the normal daily recycling load. This can drive the amount of bilirubin into a range that requires treatment.

Fortunately, in the majority of cases, the bilirubin level in newborns is within the range of the normal expected amount and is easily dealt with by the infant's liver. This "physiologic jaundice" usually requires no treatment. If bilirubin levels reach an unacceptable level, treatment is easily and safely administered. That treatment consists of placing the infant under "the lights," known as phototherapy, usually done in the nursery of the hospital where the infant was born. Many years ago, medical researchers discovered that ultraviolet light had the ability to convert bilirubin from a toxic to a nontoxic product. The blood passing through the skin is exposed to this ultraviolet light, and bilirubin is chemically changed. The light does not excrete the bilirubin—that is a job for the liver—but it slows the rate of rise and lowers the risk of high levels of bilirubin. The level of bilirubin is controlled by phototherapy. As the liver matures, the bilirubin is excreted from the body, the level of jaundice decreases, and the treatment can be discontinued. Careful monitoring for jaundice in the newborn warns the provider when to institute this type of treatment.

Today, newborns are being discharged from hospitals after two to four days, but jaundice can appear from three to seven days. Early screening in a pediatrician's office after discharge from the hospital is the best method of identifying jaundice and treating those infants who require treatment.

Nancy's Story: My Baby Is Yellow

Having had a caesarean section for our first child, I had no choice in the matter for our second; I was an automatic candidate to deliver by C-section. In the late 1970s, ultrasound technology was just coming to the forefront, and obstetricians had a powerful new tool at their disposal. My doctor recommended that in the ninth month of pregnancy, I have an ultrasound to determine the size of the baby since I would not be going into labor. My due date was in early February, and the ultrasound was scheduled just after New Year's Day.

Primitive by today's standards, an ultrasound then was only expected to show the size of the baby, especially the size of the head; whereas today, ultrasonographers can even determine the sex of a baby. Such detail was not available in 1977. When the technician told me that my baby's head was the size of a forty-week fetus, I was stunned. I was five weeks away from my due date. The ultrasound film was read by a radiologist, who confirmed the findings. The only reasonable course of action, my doctor thought, was to split the difference and deliver the baby by C-section in the third week of January.

The second C-section was much easier than the first. I was completely rested and alert. I had no pain before delivery, and the pain afterward didn't seem as bad. I was happy to watch the evening television miniseries Roots as I was recuperating while my baby was cared for by nurses and my two-year-old was at home with her dad.

Soon after the delivery, it was clear that Matt was "on the early side." My original due date was probably the correct one; this baby had a big head like his paternal grandfather and he weighed almost eight pounds. It was not surprising that the ultrasonographers thought that he was full-term. He was also incredibly sleepy; although my milk came in on the third day, this baby was fairly disinterested. No amount of poking, prodding, and thumps on the feet could arouse him. He slumbered most of the time.

Our pediatrician was not surprised that this baby developed significant jaundice on his sixth day. His immaturity, I was told, was the issue. But we had an enormous advantage; because of my C-section, we were still in the hospital since all mothers and their babies delivered by C-section stayed in the hospital about seven days in those good ole days. The treatment was a simple matter; the lights were readied, and Matt spent the better part of the next two days under those lights.

Oh Sugar, Oh Sugar

Another chemical that is out of your control is the baby's blood sugar. The human body controls the level of blood sugar within a very narrow normal range. When the blood sugar level falls below normal, we call it hypoglycemia. Hypoglycemia is a problem because all cells of the body utilize sugar as an energy source. Prolonged periods of low blood sugar level starve cells of their energy source and can lead to unconsciousness and seizures because of inadequate fuel for brain cells. Newborns frequently experience short periods of hypoglycemia, which are well tolerated by the infant and are not dangerous. The instability of blood sugar levels in the newborn is a consequence of having spent nine months sharing a circulation with the mother. Maternal insulin crosses the placenta and controls the baby's blood sugar level. Once the umbilical cord is cut, control of a newborn's blood sugar is passed immediately onto the infant. The fine-tuning of this system commonly takes a day or two, and many of my newborn patients experience a moderate period of low blood sugar level. Despite the swings in blood sugar levels, most infants do not show any symptoms. Clearly, babies tolerate these low levels of sugar much better than adults.

Usually, the blood sugar level returns to normal over a day without having to do much. In the event that treatment is necessary, the simple response is to provide supplementary feeding of sugar.

Today's Forecast Calls for Rising or Falling Temperatures

Temperature regulation is another function that a newborn infant must learn to deal with once she is outside of the womb. We regulate our temperatures by sending out neurologic signals to blood vessels in our skin; these signals tell the blood vessels to either contract and retain heat or dilate and release heat. As with so many other neurologic systems in a baby, these pathways of communication are immature and function somewhat primitively. A baby can easily overheat if she is excessively wrapped or can lose too much heat if she is not adequately wrapped. There is no magic rule for temperature regulation, but usually the baby learns to control her temperature adequately by her second day.

Just Watch Those Ounces Melt Away

Finally, let's review weight or the loss thereof. All babies lose weight just after birth. They actually lose approximately 10 percent of their weight during the first week of life. This weight loss is normal during this time as the infant is merely urinating off excess fluid. When I do my rounds on newborns, I am bewildered at the number of nurses who are focused on every ounce of weight lost. I encourage nurses to look at the baby rather than the weight chart. If a baby is really losing excess weight and becoming dehydrated, then her respiratory rate and heart rate will increase, and she may appear to be floppy and lacking in muscle tone. Most infants I see, who have supposedly lost "too much" weight, appear perfectly healthy, with normal heart rates and unlabored breathing. Weight, like many other factors we can measure, needs to be evaluated in the context of the entire picture. Most infants who are in trouble due to excessive weight loss will exhibit a constellation of symptoms.

What to Know about the Second and Third Days

It is very important to realize that your newborn baby is still making major adjustments to extra-uterine life. The cardiovascular system is still making transitions. The liver is immature and is just beginning to crank out the enzymes that break down nutrients and detoxify waste materials. The central and peripheral nervous systems are trying to fine-tune body temperature regulation. The endocrine system is beginning to assume control of blood sugar levels as well as maintenance of metabolic stability.

To observers, the baby seems to be sleeping (almost too much!), but actually she is working like crazy to bring various bodily systems up to speed. The calmness on the outside belies the frenetic pace of adjustments occurring on the inside. Just a day or two earlier, her mother handled these life-supporting tasks for her fetus as well as for herself. Just as a mother's body now makes adjustments to sustain only one living being, her newborn is making adjustments too. As noted earlier, these first few days were meant for you to hold and admire the fruits of your labor.

- Jaundice is a physiologic occurrence that is affected by many factors. It is very common and easily treated if necessary.

- Hypoglycemia (low blood sugar) is well tolerated by most infants but must be monitored and evaluated since the causes are many.

- Fluid loss and, therefore, weight loss are normal physiologic occurrences in new babies.

- Heart murmurs come and go in newborns as they undergo transition to extra-uterine life. Those murmurs are common and usually benign.

- Temperature instability is another control issue that relates to immature regulatory mechanisms in the newborn, and it is usually self-limited.

9

Preemptive Advice: Learn What to Expect in the Next Few Weeks

It is reported in the Bible that "he rested on the seventh day from all his work which he had made." On the seventh day, new mothers will not begin resting from all the work that they have made. In fact, by day seven, all of an infant's systems are full steam ahead. The heart and lungs have settled into their roles to provide oxygen and nutrition to all the tissues of the baby. The infant's kidneys are, at this point, able to deal with excretion and maintenance of fluid balance. The endocrine system has kicked in, and it maintains blood sugar levels and regulates metabolic balance. The gastrointestinal tract and liver are now prepared to absorb food and process that food into energy calories to build new tissues and increase the size of other tissues. The same gastrointestinal, renal, and respiratory systems are capable of processing waste products and excreting toxins, unwanted metabolites, and nonessential nutrients out of the body. All body systems are incredibly busy during the first week in preparation to assume the tasks of growth. The only systems that view day seven as a day of rest are the neurologic and the muscular systems. These two systems will remain immature in their development for quite a while. The brain is content to respond to pain, discomfort, or hunger with the simple actions of sucking and crying. And full-time sucking begins to happen on day seven.

Every Day Another Sucker Is Born

Day seven marks the beginning of the greatest period of growth any child will ever experience. In just three hundred and sixty-five days, he would have grown about ten inches and put on about fourteen pounds. When I talk about growth in actual quantity, that growth does not seem very dramatic. But what if I say that a baby has a 30 percent increase in height and a 150 percent increase in weight in just one year? Imagine if this rate of growth occurred within one year to an average adult, that adult would then be about sixteen feet tall and weigh 520 pounds. When I relate this information to patients, they invariably say, "You've got to be kidding, Dr. Heller." The rate of growth in a baby's first year is truly phenomenal.

Fill Her up with High Test; We Got Places to Go

This rapid growth requires energy, and the source of the energy is either breast milk or formula. milk. The baby determines the frequency of the fill-ups. Just as a locomotive going full speed requires a coalman to keep filling the engine with fuel, so too a newborn needs frequent refueling to achieve maximal growth. Because of this rapid growth rate, an infant needs to feed every three hours. At the end of the first week, breasts have about one ounce of breast milk between them. At two weeks, the breasts have about two ounces; and at three weeks, about three ounces.

Babies suck for both the acquisition of nutrients as well as for comfort and pleasure. Because they need to suck beyond their need for food, babies suck much longer than it takes them to empty the breast of fluid. Within fifteen to twenty minutes, the breasts are empty, but an infant will continue to suck for twice that time for comfort and pleasure. Usually, formula-fed babies chow down considerably more than they need because they will continue to suck for pleasure but continue to receive milk.

This rapid rate of growth in the first year does not occur evenly over the entire year. An average baby will gain 5.5 pounds in the first three months, 4 pounds between three and six months, 3 pounds between six and nine months, and 2 pounds from nine months to a year. In other words, our speeding locomotive is actually slowing down over the first year, and the refueling needs are also decreasing as time goes on. Basically, babies' initial growth in the first months of the first year far exceeds that of growth in the later months of the first year. Thus, the frequency of feeding early in the first year is more than later in the first year. A newborn needs to feed about every three to four hours to grow well. Between three and four months old, a baby can sleep at night for eight hours because his growth rate has slowed significantly. Daytime feedings alone become adequate to meet energy needs after three months of age.

A Day of Rest

This fact has great relevance for a nursing or formula-feeding mother. Frequently, I am asked by a new mother, "When can I expect the baby (and as a corollary herself) to sleep through the night?" I reply that a good night's sleep will happen at about three months. My statement fits with our scientific data. Newborns, studied at various ages by electroencephalograms to judge brain activity and by blood tests of serotonin, melotonin, and steroid levels to determine day/night variations, all show that day/night integration in infants is not established until about three months of age.

Thus, with biblical phraseology, I can predict, "She rested on the ninetieth day from all her work which she had made." Ninety days is a long time, but the reward of a full night's sleep is incredible.

I will never forget the mix of joy and fear in Nancy's face when we awoke one day after a full night's sleep. We were joyful that we had slept a whole night and fearful that something must be wrong. "Did you get up and take care of Marissa!" "No, I thought you did." We both dashed to the nursery with its playful animal wallpaper and apprehensively peered into the fabric-lined white crib. Marissa was fast asleep and breathing steadily. We could hardly believe we had survived to this moment. Marissa could actually sleep through the night. This was a major neurological event in her life and a wonderful uplifting event for us. Marissa's locomotive was beginning to slow down. The need to refuel every three hours with calories had come to an end for Marissa, and our fear that we would never sleep again had been proven to be unfounded.

Never Trust a Magic Number

I have the great fortune of taking care of many patients and families. I know babies who are doing fine, getting into a sleep pattern at two months, and some who take longer. Three months seem a reasonable expectation. Certainly, under three months of age, our scientific measurements show that a baby is not expected to sleep for prolonged periods. Patterned sleep behavior does not usually occur until three months of age. A baby who will not sleep eight hours at night after three months is pushing the normal biologic limits for this behavior.

Every grandma, grandpa, and medical student knows that babies walk at one year of age. But that's not quite true. After all, some babies walk when they are younger than twelve months. I do not become concerned if a baby is not walking at fourteen or fifteen months of age. At that point in time, if he does not walk and the rest of his exam is normal, I encourage his parents not to pick him up. If he is challenged, will he step up to the plate and accomplish the task? Only if he fails this challenge will I send him to a neurologist or orthopedist for evaluation.

I approach the behavioral development of a baby's sleep pattern in the same way. A baby under three months of age is presumed to be neurologically immature and unable to sleep for seven or eight hours at night. However, after three months of age, it is reasonable to challenge that baby. I advise parents not to peek in every three or four hours and give the baby a chance to figure out how to put himself to sleep. This is not unfair to the baby. By refraining from picking their baby after three or four hours, parents help figure out whether their baby has a problem or not and whether that problem is worth pursuing.

There Is Light at the End of the Tunnel, but What Is in the Tunnel?

For most babies, three months represents the light at the end of the tunnel. That is when parents get some sleep and start feeling like humans again. The days and weeks leading up to three months also have a certain predictability. Part of pre-emptive medicine is to be aware of these predictable factors and behaviors. If you know what to expect, you are not surprised, and you are prepared to respond appropriately. Among those behaviors that are definitely predictable is the amount of crying time that babies experience in a day. Most likely, your baby will begin to cry for three hours a day somewhere between two and four weeks of age and will continue this behavior until he is eight to twelve weeks of age. As with many behavioral and developmental issues, we do not understand why this happens, but we know that it does happen. The three hours of crying tend to bunch together in the evenings. The first two weeks are relatively easy compared to the later period from two weeks to three months. In the first week, babies sleep 70 percent of the time. During the second week, that number falls to about 50 percent of the time. Beginning with the third week, sleep time tends to fall dramatically. Unfortunately, the decrease in sleep time overlaps the increase in crying time. Knowing how predictable this crying is does not tell us what causes it. Many give it the name colic, but that is not an accurate answer (see chapter on colic).

Wow! That Is One Ugly-looking Baby

On top of the increase in crying time, beginning at two to three weeks of age, babies begin to break out with facial rashes and blotchy skin. As luck would have it, not only is the baby crying more, but he is also becoming blemished. At birth, any baby has full-blown levels of hormones just like an adult female. Your baby has spent the last nine months within your womb and is chemically a woman. This is true whether the baby is a boy or a girl. When hormone levels, either high or low, are stable, the skin is usually in great shape. During periods when hormones are falling or rising rapidly, the skin may break out with acne, like lesions. In adolescents, hormones are rising and unstable, and acne is a common problem. After birth, the baby's hormones are falling and unstable, and acne is also a problem. In most cases, babies between two and twelve weeks of age have a face only a mother could love. If you are the mother, you will find it difficult to love a pimply faced person who cries three hours every evening. And to top it off, I have more bad news.

Smile though Your Heart Is Breaking

If crying for three hours and having a terrible complexion were not bad enough, we can add one more blow to your relationship with your new baby; babies don't smile for the first few weeks. Nancy and I remember very well how down we felt before our baby smiled at us. A genuine smile from a baby is a terrific reward for a new mother. A smile means that your baby recognizes you and is pleased. In a nonverbal relationship, a smile replaces words and conveys so many unsaid feelings, including "Thank you," "You're a great mom," and "I love you too." Crying is viewed as the registering of a complaint; smiling is viewed as the acknowledgement of a job well done. Unfortunately, newborn babies do not smile until about six weeks of age. Six weeks is a long time to wait for a thank you, but wait you must. Dealing with a pimply faced, complaining, unsmiling person is no one's idea of a fun time. But like much of behavioral development in children, this first six-week period is well defined and has little or nothing to do with you personally.

Boys Will Be Boys, Girls Will Be Girls, and Amazingly, Babies Will Be Babies

Basically, a baby's neurological development is programmed in a rather predictable manner. The inability to sleep for long periods has nothing to do with you. The failure to smile should not be taken personally. For that matter, his acne is not your fault. I know, when we had our first child, we were endlessly trying to figure out what we had done wrong. We tried to determine why we could not get our child to sleep or seem happy. We, somehow, were under the misconception that our baby's behavior was all about us. We did not understand that, in fact, infant behavior is all about the baby. This may not sound very intelligent, but in retrospect, I learned that the baby was being a baby. The inability to accept that a baby following these definable patterns of behavior was simply being a baby has lead to alternative answers. Doctors have put the label of colic or milk intolerance or gastroesophogeal reflux disease on what is predictable and normal behavior.

So What Can I Do?

Accepting that babies can be predictably miserable is helpful. Do not feel angry or frustrated with your newborn. His behavior is normal for his age. Do not feel like a failure or unloved. The baby is acting in accordance with well-known developmental patterns. Many people find that taking a walk or a drive in a car reduces the baby's fussy periods. Most babies respond to being swaddled tightly and put down. They seem to want less handling rather than more. I know that one "cure" does not fit all, but you don't have to invent a diagnosis to define the condition. The condition is normal.

- Be prepared for a lot of sleepless periods that may appear to have no rewards.

- As always, get rest when you can, and don't take your baby's behavior personally.

- Patience is a virtue. Many baby behaviors are patterned and predictable.

10

The First Visit in a Pediatrician's Office

I will forever remember the first newborn I cared for in the hospital. Henry was born at the old Boston Lying-In Hospital, and in those days, as a perfectly well newborn, he "laid-in" for four days. When I discharged him from the hospital, I gave his mom instructions on how to care for his umbilical cord and what to do to help his circumcision to heal. She then asked me a simple question, "When do I come to see you?" I was stupefied. In fact, I was doubly stupefied.

First, I could not believe that she wanted to come to the office and see me. I was a newly practicing pediatrician, having spent the prior three years at the Massachusetts General Hospital. During my residency and fellowship in nephrology, the hospital had not focused at all on primary care. When I decided to become a practicing pediatrician, I had expected to have, for at least the first several months, the close guidance and attention of the very experienced and excellent pediatrician whom I was joining. But that was not to be the case because his heart condition forced him to take a medical leave, and I was thrust into a role that I was unprepared for. New at providing advice, I was fumbling for the right answers during Henry's hospital stay. So, of course, I was pleased, and also stunned, that this mother wanted me to be her son's pediatrician.

Secondly, I was also astonished because I had no clue when the first in-office appointment should be. I actually did not know what to tell her. Most young hospital-based pediatricians in the 1970s were not taught how to practice primary care or how to provide continuity of care. Instead, we advised patients to call a "real" pediatrician for follow-ups. Not having practiced in an office yet, I was not yet a "real" pediatrician.

Luckily, I knew how to think fast on my feet. After all, I had graduated from one of the country's best programs. I could diagnose rare disorders and save lives. Surely, I should be able to deal with this dilemma. The best answer I could think of was to tell her that my secretary would call her with some open appointment times. My answer was disingenuous; since I was just beginning my practice, I had no patients booked for the entire year!

However, my plan worked like a charm. While I am sure that she saw through my subterfuge, Henry's mom was gracious enough to accept my answer, and she agreed to wait for a call from my secretary. I immediately rushed to the hospital bedside of my mentor and asked him when to schedule the first in-office follow-up exam on newborns. His body language conveyed that he thought I was an idiot; he rolled his eyeballs and said, "Three weeks, of course. Didn't they teach you anything at Mass. General?" I realized that even though Henry's mom had confidence in me, my new boss was definitely developing some doubts.

Infants Have More Frequent Office Visits Today

Today, most pediatricians see newborns for a full visit by two weeks of age, not three. (And most pediatricians see newborns for a quick check for jaundice within a few days of discharge from the hospital.) But in the 1970s and 80s, managed care had not pressured doctors and hospitals to release newborns after two days in the hospital. Twenty-five years ago, babies remained in the hospital until the potential for jaundice had subsided or declared itself in which case treatment was begun and hospital stays were extended. Hospitals had not pressured mothers to breast-feed before they are physiologically able. And new mothers who were not subjected to these pressures had confidence that they could do what their mothers and grandmothers and great-grandmothers did—breast-feed successfully.

A Weighty Issue: Three Weeks Is a Magic Number

But why was a three-week visit the magic number twenty-five years ago? The reason that we examined newborns at three weeks old was their weight. Babies lose 10 percent of their weight in the first seven to ten days. That 10 percent is in part the extra fluid that had been in their lungs. Since they are no longer floating in amniotic fluid, they pee that fluid off and, consequently, lose weight. After that initial weight loss, babies will begin to gain weight at about one ounce (thirty grams) each day.

New Math—Definitely Not Rocket Science

What will a typical seven-pound-eight-ounce (7 lbs, 8 oz) baby weigh at one, two, and three weeks of age?

1. Calculate the initial weight loss. A 10 percent weight loss for a seven-pound-and-eight-ounce baby is twelve ounces (12 oz).

2. Subtract that weight loss number of twelve ounces from the seven-pound-and-eight-ounce birth weight. At one week old, our baby should weigh six pounds and twelve ounces (6 lbs 12 oz). This takes into account the fact that breast-fed babies get very little milk in the first week.

3. Add in the amount of gain (seven days x one ounce per day—do not count the first seven days of the baby's life). At two weeks old, the baby would have gained an ounce a day or seven ounces. Add this to the one week weight of six pounds and twelve ounces. Thus, at two weeks, our baby will weigh seven pounds and three ounces (7 lbs 3 oz). STOP! Think about that. At two weeks old, a normal baby is NOT back to his birth weight.

4. Add the gain of seven ounces to the two-week weight of seven pounds and three ounces. Yikes, our baby now weighs seven pounds and ten ounces (7 lbs 10 oz)! Our baby has finally, at THREE weeks old, barely surpassed her birth weight. At three weeks old, our baby is a mere two ounces more than her weight on the day she was born. Pause and ponder that fact for a moment. All of those worries such as "Is the baby growing?" "Is my milk in?" and "Am I making enough milk?" are not worth the worry. Realize that the answer does not come for three weeks. That is why, in the "old days," our first in-office examination of your baby did not occur until three weeks after birth. At three weeks old, if the baby had reached or exceeded her birth weight, we knew all was well. If the baby was below birth weight, we knew there was a problem.

The Rules Changed, but the Reality Did Not

Rules about the frequency of office visits began to change about fifteen years ago. Pediatricians began to see newborns for office exams at two weeks of age. Many very good reasons exist for this change. If babies are failing to thrive for heart, lung, or nutritional reasons, a pediatrician can begin to treat these problems sooner than later. We can advise parents about what changes to expect as the baby enters its huge growth surge. We can begin immunization against hepatitis B.

Unfortunately, the notion that babies reach birth weight at the first visit was not adjusted for the fact that the first visit was now a week earlier. Both doctors and parents began to assume that the baby would have gained enough to return to birth weight at the second-week checkup. While this was true for the three-week visit as noted above, it was definitely not true for the two-week visit.

All too often, I become involved with patients who come to us from other practices because their children are diagnosed as failing to thrive. I find it tragic when I work through the numbers; in most cases, these babies had perfectly normal weight loss and were perfectly normal below-birth-weight babies at two weeks old. Yet the message to the mothers of these babies is that mom's breast milk is inadequate, and she must either give up nursing or supplement feedings with formula; we push moms to make milk quickly (which no mother can physiologically do), and then we cause them to feel like failures when the baby is not at birth weight at two weeks (which some babies cannot physiologically do). The tragedy is that too many moms surrender to these pressures and stop breast-feeding their babies altogether.

Problems: Who's Got Problems?

Compare breast-feeding capabilities with realistic information about what to expect for weight gain. Clearly, most moms and babies are doing very well. The current medical advice to push for unattainable lactation in the first days and our incorrect expectation for babies to gain weight quickly are the real problems. We seem to be on a quest to find diseases and disorders where they do not exist. Too often, our focus is on illness and not on understanding wellness.

The bottom line is that both lactation and initial weight gain take more time than our current guidelines allow. Women lactate and babies grow no differently today than they did thousands of years ago. The failure to gain enough weight to reach birth weight by two weeks is not a problem for the baby or the mother; such "failure" is only a problem manufactured by the medical system.

Today's First Well Visit Is at Two Weeks

For many new parents, the trip to the doctor's office for the two-week visit may be the first time that they have left the house with their newborn (other than the trip home from the hospital and the trip to the pediatric office to have the baby's jaundice level checked). When parents arrive with their new baby for the two-week visit, they invariably arrive a bit late and usually are carrying enough equipment to support triplets. At times, it appears that they are prepared to stay overnight! I wonder how long they envision they would be staying in the office. The amount of equipment they carry is amazing. Amidst an array of diaper bags, hospital medical records, nursing supplies, supplemental formula, and extra clothing, all heaped in a huge carriage, I am delighted to find a baby scrunched contentedly in a combination car seat/infant carrier. After struggling with the car seat safety buckle and after removing multiple layers of unnecessary clothing, we find a two-week-old infant, usually sleeping contentedly. But this baby now looks significantly different from how she looked on her first day of life.

What to Expect at the Two-week Visit

Having finally undressed the baby and stored all his paraphernalia, we get down to business. Before I put a baby on the scale, I work out what I expect the baby's weight would be. I subtract 10 percent of his birth weight and then add an ounce for each day of life since the seventh day. In the vast majority of cases, the baby has gained the weight that I have calculated; rarely, I do find a baby who has not.

For those babies who are below weight expectations, the most common reason is that the mother has been subjected to so many different opinions about feeding that her anxiety and stress levels have affected her milk production. Before you get caught in this trap, ask yourself the following questions: Did your mother nurse you? Did her mother nurse her? Did your great-grandmother nurse your grandmother? The answer to at least one of those questions has to be YES. From that point backward to the beginning of life on earth, the answer has to be YES. Now turn that thought around. Clearly, you come from a family that has successfully breast-fed its babies for thousands of years. Your family and ancestral history of successful breast-feeding is not an unusual history. Were it otherwise, you and many others would not be here today. I often think that the less advice moms hear about breast-feeding, the better and easier the process would be for them.

Turn Water to Milk: Rest and Don't Stress

When a baby is below the second-week weight expectations, I encourage breast-feeding moms to review what is happening in their lives. What stresses are interfering with their production of milk? Are they doing chores when the baby is sleeping? Are they food shopping, laundering clothes, making meals, and entertaining family and friends? Are they fretting about other issues in their lives? How much liquid are they consuming? As said in the chapter on breast-feeding, milk production increases if mom is rested, unstressed, and drinks large quantities of water. I encourage moms to try that approach before giving up nursing and to schedule another visit within a few days to check on the baby's weight.

A Two-week-old Loses Its Newborn Status

By two-weeks old, the baby's skin has taken a dramatic downward turn. The slow disappearance of maternal hormones causes infant rashes, which are essentially acne. Baby's hands, legs, and feet have significant peeling of the skin. Remember how your fingertips seemed to take on a wrinkled appearance and odd feeling after sitting in a bathtub for a long time. Imagine spending nine months in that bathtub. The baby spent the last nine months floating in the water of the womb and is now undergoing transition to an entirely new environment. That transition is characterized by the shedding or peeling of the skin that formerly was endlessly moistened.

Even Baby Boys Have Breasts?

Another difference from birth is the development of breast tissue in both girl and boy babies who are breast-fed. If I squeeze the nipples of a two-week-old, I will often cause the expulsion of milk. The well-known fact that infants produce milk has the common name "witches' milk." Milk and breast engorgement in the baby are wonderful signs that nursing is going well. Having spent nine months inside full-fledged, hormonally balanced women, all newborns, either gender, are born with the hormones of full-fledged, hormonally balanced women.

Breast-fed babies obtain lactating hormones from mom's breast milk, and the consequence is that the babies can make milk and their nipples become engorged. The engorgement can only occur if breast-feeding is working normally. This breast engorgement will decrease and disappear over the ensuing weeks as the baby loses those adult female hormone levels and, therefore, will no longer respond to the lactating hormone.

No More Cone Heads

A baby's skull is usually dramatically different by two weeks of age. During birth, the pushing of the infant's head down the cervical canal causes considerable molding of the skull. Most babies are born with "cone heads". At two weeks old, the bony plates are moving back and rounding off.

No More Umbilical Cord

Also, at two weeks old, the cord is usually gone and the belly button should be dry. If it is not gone or there is moist granulation tissue at the umbilical site, your doctor will cauterize the cord, a fairly common procedure that is not a significant problem.

On the other hand, the issue of whether the baby's belly button is an innie or an outie is a big deal for some parents. If the bellybutton is extruded, that extrusion has nothing to do with your obstetrician or whoever cut the cord. The umbilical cord dries up first from the point of cutting back toward the infant's body. Nature determines how far back this drying will happen. Most protruding umbilical stumps are actually due to the baby's lack of abdominal muscles. As infants mature, most belly buttons become perfectly normal looking by three years of age.

A Full Physical at Every Well Visit

At every well visit, a pediatrician will examine your baby from head to foot and front to back; anomalies may appear over time. Hearts and hips will be rechecked; any "defects" noticed by parents will be examined and explained.

Preemptive Medicine Advice

Your baby will now enter what many call the colicky or fussy phase of infancy. You are about to enter the twilight zone. As explained in more detail in the chapter on colic, babies seem programmed to have three hours of crying each day between the second and up to the twelfth week of life.

Also, dads become a bit "colicky" after two weeks of mom's breast-feeding. Dads want to care for their newborns as much as moms. I felt frustrated that, whenever my babies were crying, all I could say was "What you want, I haven't got, so here is your mother." I felt happier when I could feed my baby too. A bit of diluted juice or Nancy's pumped breast milk in a bottle enabled me to share in the nurturing process and gave Nancy some needed rest.

- Your baby should be back to birth weight by three weeks old, not two weeks old!

- If your breast-fed baby is not meeting weight expectations using the formula above, rest more, drink more water, and try not to feel stressed.

- At two weeks old, babies have rashes and peeling skin.

- At two weeks old, all babies, boy or girl, have breasts, and some even make milk.

- At two weeks old, baby heads and cords look much better.

11

Colic, Crying, Peeing, and Pooping—the Crying or Fussy Baby

Pediatric books contain many descriptions of a colicky baby, who, at two to eight weeks old, suddenly has episodes of crying associated with pulling his legs up and pushing down. The baby appears to be having trouble with his stomach. In fact, he seems to be unsuccessful in his attempt to have a huge bowel movement. He is inconsolable. He goes back and forth to the breast or bottle, and yet no amount of feeding, patting, or rocking seems to help. These episodes usually begin in the evening and can last up to three hours. They end as abruptly as they begin, and the baby returns to his daytime pattern of behavior only to become inconsolable again the next evening. Many label this behavior as colic. Why do some babies develop colicky behavior?

A. The Mother Is to Blame

Some pediatricians and parents need a villain to blame for this infant behavior. If the mother is breast-feeding, she is told that she ate or drank some food or liquid that is making the baby "colicky." Yet only caffeine, alcohol, and some medications affect the baby; no other liquids do so. Green vegetables and beans may be blamed for increased gas in the mother. The digestion of these vegetables occurs in the mother's bowel, and the bacterial breakdown can cause increased gas production in the mom's intestine. These vegetables are part of the mother's diet. The baby's diet is breast milk. In fact, breast milk remains amazingly consistent in its content of fats, carbohydrates, proteins, and minerals despite what the mother's diet includes. Moms can eat bland or spicy food, American or Asian food, French or Mexican food; breast milk remains the same.

91

Indeed, the content of breast milk is maintained even to the detriment of the mother. For example, if a mother does not ingest enough calcium, her body will, for as long as it needs to, steal calcium from her bones to ensure an adequate amount in her breast milk. Further, the content of breast milk is the same, morning, noon, and night. If breast milk were the culprit, babies should be colicky or fussy, morning, noon, and night; yet most of babies' colic occurs only in the evenings. We absolutely should not blame a breast-feeding mother for the "colicky" behavior. Answer A is false.

B. The Formula Is to Blame

Formula-fed babies can also be colicky. Obviously, this is further evidence that mom's breast milk does not cause colic. For formula-fed babies, since we cannot blame the mother, we turn to formula as the cause of the baby's colic. Whichever formula is initially fed to a baby is both blamed and changed if that baby becomes "colicky." If the baby is being fed cow's milk-based formula, mom is told that cow's milk is making the baby "colicky" and is instructed to switch to a soy-based formula. The rationale in this scenario is that perhaps the baby is allergic to cow's milk. However, if the infant is fed soy-based formula from birth, that baby is switched on to very expensive predigested formulas to treat the "colic."

However, if both formula-fed and breast-fed babies get colic, the source of baby's nutrition is clearly not involved in the fussy behavior. In my thirty-year career, I have seen babies who exhibit colicky behavior no matter what the source of their nutrition. Whether fed with breast milk, modified cow's milk, or soy formula, the majority of babies exhibit colicky or fussy behavior. Answer B is false.

C. The Gas Is to Blame

Others cast the blame on public enemy number one, gas, whether baby is burping or farting. Some pediatricians prescribe medications to decrease the size of gas bubbles on the theory that a little fart or little burp is better than a big fart or big burp.

Amazingly, gas plays a major role in an infant's life, even beyond colic. Parents call frequently with questions about gas; they believe that gas is causing their baby's fussiness. At the two-month visit, when I ask, "Did your baby smile?" many parents tell me that the baby smiled, but they think the smiling was caused by "gas." Somehow, we are expected to believe that gas is responsible both for making babies fussy and, at the same time, making them smile. My medical training did not prepare me for this juxtaposition.

One's life experience provides some answers to this conundrum. On first dates, at weddings, and at bar mitzvahs, I had pains as I resisted my desire to let gas out. On the other hand, when alone in the front seat of the car or walking outdoors, I didn't force myself to hold gas in and had no pain as a result. But when I had an abdominal flu, I suffered abdominal pains whether passing gas or not, and I had no desire to eat. Finally, I recall an embarrassing moment at a wedding as I unintentionally passed some gas when laughing at a guest's very funny joke.

Do these situations apply to a newborn? Babies certainly aren't worried about social conventions; they don't control pee and poop and aren't holding in their gas either. Clearly, gas cannot be hurting babies on the basis of holding gas in, since they don't perform this socially correct behavior.

Could the baby have a flu or stomach virus as the cause of the gas and colicky behavior? Yes, but in that situation, that infant will have fever, decreased fluid intake, and begin to look ill, which is not the case with the vast majority of fussy or colicky babies, who are happy to keep feeding despite their gas. Secondly, no baby has daily bouts of stomach virus only in the evenings for several weeks.

The truth is that we all have gas in the rectums of our colons all of the time. Gas is normally created by bacteria in the process of breaking down the food in our intestines; gas exists in our rectums without causing any problems. When pressure is applied to the abdomen, gas may be extruded. A laugh, a cough, and a sneeze all cause an increase in abdominal pressure, which is what accounts for the embarrassing moment I experienced at a wedding.

Both babies and adults have the gastrocolic reflex that causes an increase in abdominal pressure. The gastrocolic reflex occurs whenever the stomach begins to fill with food. The intake of food and stretching of the stomach sends endocrine and neurologic signals to the rest of the colon to contract and prepare to empty so that the gastrointestinal system can process the next load. During every feeding, a baby normally pulls up his legs and presses down to encourage the lower colon to empty. Even if there is no stool in the rectum, the baby will go through these normal motions. The increase in pressure may cause gas to be expelled. The bottom (excuse the double entendre) line is that you do not either create or control gas, nor does it bother the baby unless he is sick with a virus or flu. Gas is an innocent bystander waiting harmlessly until the "wind" is knocked out. A laugh, a cough, a sneeze, or a feeding all trigger a rise in abdominal pressure that expels the gas. Answer C is false.

D. The Reflux Is the Culprit

The latest culprit is gastroesophogeal reflux disorder (GERD). Basically, acid reflux is blamed as the cause of the "colic" on the theory that acid backs up into the baby's esophagus and causes discomfort. Our radiological technologies clearly demonstrate that this reflux of stomach contents in babies occurs. Those who subscribe to this theory may choose a combination of a medication to decrease acid secretion and a special infant position during feeding to decrease the reflux. But, as stated in the chapter on GERD, gastroesophogeal reflux is normal in all babies until they are about ten months old whether they have colic or not. While gastroesophogeal reflux disorder sounds impressive and is a mouthful, GERD is not the cause of colic. Answer D is false.

E. "Colic" Is *Normal*

Now we have our lineup of suspects. Not surprisingly, they are the usual suspects we vilify whenever we are unhappy with infant behavior: the mother, the formula, the gas, and the reflux. You can easily choose one as the cause of colicky and fussy babies and then choose a corresponding treatment for that cause. But the correct answer is E, "none of the above."

Colicky behavior is normal, for both boys and girls, between two and eight weeks of age. Pediatric developmentalists have videotaped babies around the clock in order to define how much normal babies sleep, eat, and cry, and they have well documented the fact that normal infants cry three out of twenty-four hours between the age of two and eight weeks. The majority of this crying is in the form of inconsolable behavior for two or three hours, especially in the evening.

So what is the disease? Study after study of colic has shown that the colons of colicky babies are perfectly normal despite the fact that the word *colic* refers to the colon. Colicky babies also have normal livers and normal digestive tracts. Studies have demonstrated that the hearts, lungs, kidneys, and heads are also all normal. The truth is that colic is not an indication of any abnormality in a baby.

The Preemptive Message

We need no suspects, and we need no cures. What we need to realize and expect is that many infants cry for long periods in the evening when they are two to eight weeks old, a behavior that has been erroneously named colic. While true "colic" does not affect all babies, most babies are, at the very least, fussy and inconsolable, especially in the evening.

Let's fast forward a moment in order to put colic in perspective. When two-year-olds fall on the floor and rant and rave for thirty minutes, parents and pediatricians have a satisfactory label: the terrible twos or two-year-old tantrums. No one calls 911; no one rushes to the emergency room; no one heads to a pharmacy for medication; and no one feeds that child soy for dinner.

We do not fully understand what triggers such behavior, but we are all willing to accept it as just that—behavior. "Colic" is just another patterned behavior. Unfortunately, as the first very annoying behavior that parents encounter, colic is blown out of proportion; parents are not prepared to deal with inconsolable crying or fussiness.

Health-care providers are altogether too quick to treat colic as a disease rather than a behavioral phase. To explain that colic is normal may be a time-consuming process. Rather, the quick response is that colic is a treatable disorder. Thus, a market has sprung up for multiple new formulas and multiple medications to reduce baby gas and acid.

Unfortunately, there are side effects to this rapid approach. Mothers of three-year-olds who have had a stomachache tell me, "Oh, she was colicky as an infant and has had something wrong with her stomach since birth." Imagine thinking that your child has some chronic, underlying illness when nothing had been wrong.

Furthermore, the medications themselves, like all medicines, can have adverse effects. Even formula changes may not be totally benign. Recent reports in the *New England Journal of Medicine* suggest that the increased incidence of peanut allergy may relate to soy oils in soy milk given to infants as a "cure" for colic. The medicalization of normalcy comes with some collateral damage.

Rarely, a baby may exhibit colicky behavior that lasts well beyond three hours per day. Twice in my career, I cared for infants with severe digestive problems requiring the use of very specialized formulas. These two infants were not only colicky but were not also thriving and growing. Their failure to grow resulted in their need for a thorough evaluation and for very specialized formulas. Their prolonged crying was not the catalyst for these medical interventions; rather, the failure to thrive was.

I have found that the Boy Scouts' motto "Be Prepared" is the best "cure" for colic. Parents who know that infants will cry for up to three hours, pull up their legs, and cry or be fussy in the evening do not have to run out for medications or medical advice. The not-so-amazing fact about colic is that by three months of age, all babies are "cured." Whether one uses changes in feeding position, changes in formula, changes in mom's diet, or introduction of medications, all of these babies "recover." The obvious reason for recovery is that babies are behaving normally, without disorders or diseases in the first place.

Sleep-deprived Parents Can Lose Control

Danger does lurk here however. Colic occurs just at the time when parents are deprived of sleep; their usual daily cycle has been turned upside down since the birth of their baby. Especially because of fatigue, a parent can easily become frustrated and angry when a baby cries or fusses inconsolably. Rocking, feeding, patting, jiggling, swaying, singing, and soothing words make no difference. How frustrating! Anger and rage build up, and a parent may be tempted to shake his or her baby in a vain attempt to stop the crying. That is the worst action to take because the shaking can cause severe, irreversible brain damage as the brain is knocked inside the skull from side to side.

Crying Is Not Harmful

The best course of action is to allow the baby to cry. After changing his diaper, feeding him, and making sure that he is not otherwise ill with a fever, place him in his crib or bassinet to permit the baby to work out his issues by himself. As with older children, and even adults, crying does release tensions, and one can feel better after a good cry. Some pediatric developmentalists point out that rocking, patting, jiggling, and swaying are actions that over-stimulate babies' nervous systems, thereby worsening the colicky or fussy condition. Again, the remedy is to allow the baby to be alone, to have some time without external stimuli.

Co-Sleeping is not Worth the Risk

Do not be tempted to have your young infant sleep with you in your bed. The danger of infant suffocation is a real one, especially when you are exhausted and may sleep deeply, unaware of the danger.

Burping: Is It Necessary?

Burping is an activity that we all do with our babies. As every reader knows, burping affects both infants and adults. We all swallow air when we eat and drink; this air does not travel all the way to our rectums but comes back up as a belch or burp. Many parents attribute the fussiness of their babies to the need to be burped. Many parents think that burping is a problem. I have never seen any other mammal pick up its newborn and smack it on the back until a "good" burp came up. Imagine the damage a cow would do to its newborn if it tried this procedure. For that matter, imagine the results if an elephant tried this maneuver. Why is it necessary that humans engage in burping our infants if no other mammal seems to require this intervention? The answer is simple: we don't. This is not to say that it isn't fun and cuddly, but we really do not have to burp our babies. On many occasions, parents will hear their baby burp all by himself in his crib without any intervention from adults. That independent burp should convince parents that babies can burp all by themselves. Burping is like peeing, pooping, and farting; babies have no social control and do these bodily functions as they need to.

As noted above, sometimes, patting to encourage burping may add to a baby's crying by over-stimulating his immature nervous system. Recently, a dad described to me his situation. He spent an hour walking and patting his baby in the middle of the night because his baby had not burped. Finally, completely exhausted, he placed his baby in the crib; as he left the room, he heard a marvelous big burp. Had he only put his baby to sleep an hour earlier, perhaps he would have saved himself a great deal of frustration and gained a precious hour of sleep.

Poop: Stop Counting

A baby's bowel movements are the object of too much attention and focus. Given our national obsession about baby poops, it is no surprise that one of the biggest problems in pediatrics is encopresis in older children. Encopresis is the condition in which children retain their feces; encopresis clinics spend many dollars and hours working with stool-retaining children. Our national focus begins in the newborn nursery; every nursing shift notes how much pee and how many poops each baby made. The poops are described in terms of color, consistency, and amount. The first few bowel movements have considerable medical significance; from a medical standpoint, we are confirming that the gastrointestinal tract is patent. Beyond that, further quantification and reporting is not necessary.

While babies may push after each feeding due to the gastrocolic reflex, no one, including babies, must have a bowel movement each and every day. In fact, many infants, especially breast-fed ones, do not. The important criteria is not how frequent or even how much. Obstipation, which means infrequent stools, is not a problem as long as the stool is soft; in that case, babies can poop once every eight days or eight times in one day, and no one should be concerned.

On the other hand, if a baby's stool is hard (firmer than toothpaste), he may have constipation, which means hard stools. A baby could poop four times in a day; if those stools are all hard, he is constipated. Constipation in a baby refers to the consistency of the stool, not the frequency. Only rarely is a breast-fed baby constipated although breast-fed babies are commonly obstipated. For formula-fed babies, constipation is more common, especially on soy-based formulas. The reason that constipation can be a concern is that hard stools can tear the rectum; rectal fissures or tears are uncomfortable for anyone, including babies. While never an emergency, parents with a constipated baby should call their pediatrician for advice about stool-softening measures.

The Color of Poop

In general, the color of a baby's poop is inconsequential. Usual colors include brown, yellow, and green. Many pediatric books advise that parents call their pediatrician if the poop is green. But this advice worries parents unnecessarily. In a healthy, happy baby, green stool is perfectly acceptable. The only time that green poop signals a problem is when a baby is ill and has a fever. In that instance, if the baby's stool is green, a bacterial infection *might* be the cause of the illness and the green poop, and that situation should be evaluated by the pediatrician. When the baby's poop is black, parents should seek medical care. Black poop might be an indication of blood in the stool, and this condition should also be evaluated. Finally, if a baby has a stool with red streaking or overt blood, a call to the pediatrician is warranted.

Pee: Start Counting

The frequency of urine, on the other hand, is very important. Normal urination signifies that the baby is well hydrated and receiving adequate nutrition. "When did the baby pee last?" That is one of the first questions that any pediatrician will ask when a parent calls about an infant fever or other illness.

Under four months old, a baby should pee approximately every four hours. Infant kidneys perform a remarkable job at maintaining fluid balance. When the infant's body does not have enough fluid, the kidneys respond by retaining as much fluid as possible. After four hours, lack of urine may be a sign of dehydration and requires immediate attention.

A Pediatrician's Tough Task

One of the most difficult tasks is to convince parents that behaviors and functions such as colic, infant fussiness, gas, reflux, and infrequent bowel movements are normal. We spend far too much time focusing on what is wrong when nothing is. Unfortunately, some health-care providers are very quick to prescribe a surefire remedy rather than take the time to explain how natural these behaviors and functions are. I cringe when families new to my practice tell me how their child was "always" colicky or gassy or irritable as an infant and remains so. My observation is that if health-care providers label a normal function as a problem, that labeling affects the long-term perception that parents have about their child.

- Most babies fuss or cry, usually in the evening.

- Mom's milk, formula, gas, and/or reflux are not the culprits.

- Colic and fussiness are normal infant behaviors, just as the terrible twos are.

- Frequency of stool is not important in a normal, healthy baby.

- Frequency of pee is very important as one measure of a well-hydrated baby.

Parent Lauren R. wrote,

> *I was concerned that my infant son didn't burp easily when I patted him on the back. Dr. Dan asked me, "Have you ever been to a zoo? Have you ever seen the mother hippo burp her baby hippo?"*
>
> *Of course, I had never seen that, so I said, "No."*

Dr. Heller said, "That's because when a baby needs to burp, he generally does it on his own."

12

Four-week Visit: Anatomy of an Office Visit

What is your pediatrician thinking of at each and every regularly scheduled office visit? At a minimum, your baby is being evaluated to ensure that she is growing normally and receiving her immunizations on schedule. Parents are eager to know the height and weight. Many parents tell me that they have bets on what their baby's weight will be. Every pediatrician knows that it takes about ten minutes to accomplish this task. Undressing a baby, examining her heart, lungs, and abdomen, weighing her, and then measuring her length and head circumference are not difficult tasks. A pediatrician then plots the height and weight measurement on a chart to record visually that the baby is growing and administers the appropriate shots. In fact, to schedule your appointment and have you read and sign the HIPPA compliance forms takes longer than to perform the examination described above.

Fortunately, most pediatricians find performing this minimum evaluation both boring and unsatisfying. The great fun and excitement of being a parent or a pediatrician is not only in observing and monitoring growth but also in assessing overall development.

The Denver Developmental Assessment Scales: A Tool to Make the Complex Simple

The easiest way to assess development is to break it down into easily definable parts. From a pediatrician's point of view, four areas merit monitoring. Those areas, categorized in the Denver Developmental Assessment system, are (1) gross motor development, (2) personal-social development, (3) language development, and (4) fine motor development. The goal of this assessment is to ensure that

101

your baby is appropriately acquiring motor functions, communication abilities, and cognitive and emotional skills.

Mirror, Mirror on the Wall, Who Is the Most Developed of Them All? *Australopithecus afarensis* (Commonly Called *Homo sapiens*) Is the Winner

In medical school, I learned about normal infant and child development. After reading the first book on this subject, I wondered if I could ever be a pediatrician. I feared that I would be unable to remember the vast amount of information about motor skills and language skills. Then I read a second book which emphasized different points about development than the first book had. At that point, I went from bewildered to very confused. I stopped reading the third book midway through because I finally saw the light. Normal human development is the result of various factors and is difficult to describe in a single book.

Many pediatric books attempt to describe in detail the expected developmental milestones for any given age. This book does not. Indeed, I won't even try to rigidly describe to you a "normal" child. Development in children varies so much that, in a sense, there are no "normal" children. There are, instead, many interesting variations on "normal."

One Potato, Two Potato, Three Potato, Four

The fact is that the development of gross motor, fine motor, language, and personal-social skills depends not just on genetics but on whether you are the first, second, or third child in a family. Other factors affect development too. Are your parents teenagers or in their twenties or thirties or over forty? Is this your first marriage, or are you a single parent?

That too affects the child's development. Even if you are dealing with the firstborn baby, child development will vary with whether you are a newborn male or female, a wanted or unwanted baby, and whether your parent was a first-, second-, or third-born child in his or her own family.

Culture and language skills of the parents will also affect my description. Basically, there is no one book on the bookshelf that can tell me what your child should absolutely to be able to do or not do at any given age. Rather, my job is to figure out, overall, if your child is developing within a large range of possible behavior norms. This assessment is definitely an art and not a science. I have to meld in many factors to form a gestalt about each and every child. Assessing any child's development during a scheduled exam requires more than ten minutes and is definitely more fun and challenging than measuring and plotting the growth data and administering immunizations.

How Does Your Child Compare to My Pal Woody?

Woody is my German shorthaired pointer. His picture is on my desk, along with those of my three children. I love to look at his picture alongside my own kids and be amazed at how their developments have differed. Imagine the following, if you will. At six weeks of age, Woody could walk, run, and swim. He fed himself from a bowl and could dig and play in the yard. He was "toilet trained" in the sense that he would whine to be taken outside rather than pee or poop in his crate. He made various noises to express his needs but could not speak. He could not draw a circle.

My gaze turns to the pictures of Marissa, Matthew, and Sara. At six weeks, they did not walk, run, or swim. Nancy needs to feed them, and they do not dig and play in the yard. They are definitely not toilet trained and, in fact, seem to pee and poop on themselves with not a care in the world. One might say they are rather disgusting compared to Woody. They make various noises, but they do not speak. They cannot draw a circle. At this stage, clearly, Woody is more likely headed to Harvard, and my children are going nowhere.

What a Difference Three Years Can Make

When I compare Woody and my three children at the age of three years, the difference is astonishing. Woody is still doing what he did at six weeks of age, admittedly with more agility. He still does not talk, and he still does not draw a circle. My children, on the other hand, have caught up with Woody in the areas of walking, running, and swimming. They have come close to or attained the ability to pee and poop in the toilet rather than on themselves.

Incredibly, they have learned to draw a circle, and they have learned to talk. These are two developmental milestones that Woody will never achieve. In fact, the greatest difference between modern humans and all the other mammals is our ability to speak, and our agility with fine motor skills. The story of Woody illustrates that the most important areas of development relative to intelligence are defined by language and fine motor skills. Humans are unsurpassed in the degree that we have moved along in our manual dexterity and cognitive and communication skills.

Parents and grandparents often focus on how the child is doing relative to sitting, crawling, walking, toilet training, and behaving. Yet in the long run, the acquisition of fine motor and language skills represents a higher level of cerebral development.

Pediatric Office Visits: Much More than Just Height, Weight, and Shots

At every visit, I ask questions to determine how each child is doing in the four major areas of development. Gross motor and personal-social skills develop earlier than fine motor and language skills. While children younger than six months of age may not seem to have significant development in the four areas discussed earlier, each baby exhibits numerous tiny clues that signify the occurrence development. A smile, a laugh, a cooing sound, and a fixed stare at an object all convey pieces of information that the neuromuscular systems of the infant are becoming coordinated. Many of the chapters in this book will talk about the usual gross and fine motor, language, and personal-social skills that are expected at different ages. But that is not the whole story.

He's Got Personality: Above and Beyond the Denver Developmental Checklist

Assessing the development of any given child goes beyond the standard Denver Developmental checklist for any given age. The achievement of these developmental milestones is not written in stone. In addition to the factors of genetics, birth order, culture, and parental age, each child has his/her own distinctive personality. Personality is hard to define and wonderful to observe. We as parents try to influence our children, and children in turn try to influence their parents. Kids might choose to talk or not talk, pee or not pee, poop or not poop, sleep or not sleep, and eat or not eat. Their choices in these matters will affect their apparent developmental level. In fact, the control issues I call the slippery STEPS (sleeping, talking, eating, peeing and stooling) often influence the apparent "normal" development of a child.

The assessment of behavior and developmental level of a child at any age is complex. As much as we desire to make the complex simple, behavior and development are simply complex.

I have always been upset by calls from parents who are filled with fear and concern that their child is autistic or developmentally delayed because they read a line in a book that did not match what their child could do at a given age. All behavioral and developmental assessments must be individualized.

Whether we are talking about growth charts to assess height and weight or developmental issues, "normal" varies widely. Every child does not hit the developmental points at the exact same time. You must be open with your health care provider and vice versa about any concerns you have about issues of growth and development. In the majority of instances, parents may be worried unduly, and a pediatric healthcare provider can, and will, be able to alleviate any anxiety.

Growth Charts: Another Tool but What Do They Tell You

At each visit, your pediatrician or pediatric nurse-practitioner will plot out your baby's vital growth statistics on a growth chart. The appendix of this book includes growth charts for baby boys and baby girls from birth to thirty-six months. Those charts are also easily available on the internet. Anyone can plot the baby's length, weight, and head circumference on these charts and follow his growth progress over time. Some new parents take these charts too seriously and react fearfully if their baby's growth is consistent with the 25th percentile. If the weight percentile is below the height percentile, some parents become anxious that their baby is not gaining enough. But these charts are only tools, and many factors determine height and weight.

Tall or Small, Fat or Thin, Tell Me What Percentile I'm In

A few points about the growth chart have to be made. First, the growth chart percentiles are not percentages of the population. Rather, the numbers represent standard deviations from the norm. For example, the 50th percentile (the middle line in the chart) is the median height of the population. It does not mean that fifty out of one hundred children are on this line and have this height. Fifty out of one hundred children actually fit between the 25th percentile and the 75th percentile for height. If your child is between the 25th and 75th percentile, she has joined fifty out of one hundred kids. Basically, half the population fits between these two percentiles. Whether you are in the 25th or the 75th percentile, you are really, plus or minus, one standard deviation from the norm.

The actual height difference between the 25th and 75th percentiles is not very much.

On the other hand, the difference in inches between the 90th and 10th percentiles is more significant. Whether a child is on the 90th percentile or the 10th, he has a height that is two standard deviations from the norm. In pediatrics, a child has to fall outside two standard deviations from the norm before we can say that this child really stands out as tall or short.

Second, the growth chart is not special while your child definitely is special. Growth charts are based on a reference point for defining "normal" and that reference point is a combination of measurement results taken from a large population. The data for most of the growth charts used in the United States comes from measuring children in America who came from western European ancestries. If a baby is of Asian ancestry, she will not fit very well on these Western-derived statistics. In fact, most Chinese babies, when plotted on these charts, are at the 90th or 95th percentile during the first year of life and then seem to fall off and become smaller compared to Western infants. Similarly, if I put Western infants on a Chinese-based growth chart, they would be in the 5th to 25th percentile. The incorrect conclusion is that Chinese children are abnormally large when they are raised in America. The correct conclusion is that we are using the wrong database to measure them. Growth chart assessments, like the developmental assessments mentioned above, are influenced by many factors. In the case of growth, factors such as gestational age, ethnic background, and nutrition affect one's placement on the growth chart. The growth chart provides a framework and a general guideline, but it does not always work well for particular individuals.

Growth Charts: A Great Clinical Aid but Definitely Not the Gold Standard of Health

Growth charts are, therefore, not used as the gold standard by which to judge each child. Rather, growth charts provide information about whether your child is growing in an appropriate manner over time. Whether an individual child is large or small, consistent growth on any given percentile is the important issue. For example, if a baby's head is 25th percentile at the first checkup, that fact tells me very little. Even if the head size is 10th percentile, there is no cause for alarm. At subsequent visits, however, if the size of the head rises from the 10th to the 50th and subsequently to the 75th percentile, I will recommend an evaluation to determine if a problem exists. The head and length of a baby generally increase at a steady rate and should grow consistently along the same percentile. As with the weight, the head size or length may shift by one standard deviation up or down over time. However, if the shift becomes two standard deviations from the baseline, then a problem may indeed exist. If a baby's head has grown too fast, that fact suggests that there may be fluid on the brain rather than a great increase in brain tissue. Similarly, a length percentile that is falling by two or more standard deviations over time suggests some significant failure of growth. The cause might be metabolic, endocrine, heart, or lung disease; the growth chart does not provide the answer to that question. Rather, the growth chart provides a clue or warning that further investigation is warranted. Accurate and timely growth data is a terrific help to a pediatrician.

The Well-child Visit: The Gold Standard to Good Health

Well-child visits are scheduled in large part to coincide with the growth rate of the child. Early in infancy, growth is rapid; thus, well visits are closer together than later in infancy.

At each well-child visit, a pediatric healthcare provider (whether pediatrician or pediatric nurse-practitioner or physician assistant) combines the concrete information learned from the growth chart with the parental reports of fine motor, gross motor, language, and personal-social skills to determine how the child is developing. These visits are not just for shots. You and I want your child to become all that he or she can be, and it is the subtle findings of these early visits that can influence the outcome.

Take-home Advice at One Month of Age

A Downhill Slide for a While Tempered by a Thank-you Smile

At the four-week visit, as stated above, the growth and development of your baby will be assessed. Have no fear from the developmental point of view. Four-week-old babies do not have to do much. In fact, their major achievement at this point will be to have successfully learned how to feed well, which will be confirmed by their weight gain and growth. Seeing good growth at this juncture is a very satisfying feeling. You can be proud that you have taken the first major step toward good parenting, and that step is to provide ample nutrition for your newborn.

Despite this achievement, I have some unfortunate preemptive advice for you. Babies will continue to have an evening fussy period that usually lasts one to two hours, and this annoying behavior will continue until eight to twelve weeks of age. Babies also continue to have pimply faces due to hormones slowly disappearing. Rashes around the rectum are still common due to frequent stooling and subsequent wiping.

On the exciting side, your baby will begin to smile and make better eye contact in the next few weeks. These smiles change everything. The two-way relationship between you and your newborn is about to become more serious. Also nighttime sleep will begin to increase at roughly one additional hour more for each passing week. At the four-week visit, I am always sympathetic to how tired and worn down most parents appear to be. Luckily, at this point or sometime in the near future, babies begin to feed less frequently and sleep more as their metabolic rates begin to slow down. Soon, you will see the light at the end of the tunnel.

Relax! The Four-week Developmental Exam Is the Easiest of All

- Gross motor: Don't expect too much. Your baby may turn his head from side to side and raise it a bit when lying down. Nothing to write home about.

- Personal-social: Maybe you will see a smile, which everyone will say is due to gas. Also, you might have a three- to four-hour run of uninterrupted nighttime sleep. No guarantee.

- Language: You may notice some cooing sounds.

- Fine motor: Free pass, collect two hundred dollars. There is no fine motor development to speak of at this visit.

- Well-baby checks are wonderfully worthwhile for you and your pediatrician to ensure the normal growth and development of your baby.

Parent Victoria K. wrote,

My family is Chinese. Both of my kids have BIG heads, especially my four year old son. His head size is off the chart. Dr. Heller told me don't need to worry, Chinese babies have big heads. This is one of the funnest and truthful things someone ever said to me. My husband and I both have big heads too, so I know Dr. Heller is right.

Parent Lisa P. C. wrote,

I asked Dr. Dan if it was OK to sleep my one-month-old on her tummy, since she was female, no asthma or smokers in the family, and was therefore at very low risk for SIDS (sudden infant death syndrome). I explained that she would give us about an hour and a half of sleep on her back or six hours on her tummy. Dr. Dan grinned, and said, "The American Academy of Pediatrics strongly recommends that babies sleep on their backs" but was nodding his head 'yes' the whole time. His medical student looked appalled, but Dr. Dan said, "Sometimes the mother just knows best."

13

Pediatricks: Gastroesophogeal Reflux, a Real Trick

Some pediatricks are sleazy
When your baby upchucks and is queasy
To say this is GERD
Is truly absurd
When your infant is really just cheesy.

In 1974, Nancy and I were blessed. After a few miscarriages, we were thrilled with the birth of our first child. Soon after her birth, our enthusiasm began to sour as she began to spit up before, after, and during every feeding. Or so it seemed. My mother said, "I am not surprised that my granddaughter is a 'cheesy, yucky baby'; she is just like her father. Don't worry, she'll outgrow this by the time she is walking."

By definition, a "cheesy" baby is an infant who, during her first year of life, would throw up or calmly regurgitate part of every feeding. Usually the baby would vomit on whoever was holding her. The baby would always do this at random times. She seemed to know when you had just put away a burping towel; then she could soil your blouse or shirt directly. Rearing a "cheesy" baby was annoying and inconvenient, largely because we had to launder the baby's and our own clothes more frequently than usual. After all, no one wanted to walk around smelling like vomit.

In my own situation, by one year of age, our daughter stopped this nasty habit. The curse of the "cheesy" stomach was gone, and our laundry bill finally abated. Life in 1974 was relatively slow paced and peaceful.

My mother had provided the correct advice although she did not know the underlying reason that her son and granddaughter were "cheesy" babies. The reason is actually quite simple. A "cheesy" or "yucky" baby is normal because all newborns have immaturity, both neurological and muscular, of the gastrointestinal tract. This immaturity persists for ten months to a year.

Let's take some time to review the physiological reasons for a "cheesy" or "yucky" baby. The facts are very clear and have not changed for eons. All babies have some degree of gastroesophageal reflux (GER) because nature designed them to have GER. As an older child or adult eats, the food travels down a tube called the esophagus to the stomach. A muscle called the gastroesophogeal sphincter lies at the junction of the stomach and the esophagus. At the bottom end of the stomach lies another muscle called the pyloric sphincter, which marks the separation of the stomach and the small intestine.

Let's follow some food on its journey from a mouth to a rectum. We swallow, and food travels down into the stomach. The pyloric sphincter closes to keep the food in the stomach so the process of digestion can begin. The gastroesophogeal sphincter at the top of the stomach closes as the stomach fills up. The stomach is now closed off at the top and the bottom, forming a bag in which acid breaks down food; the stomach churns and mashes down what we have eaten. When this process is complete, the pyloric sphincter at the bottom of the stomach opens, and the stomach forcefully contracts. The churned up, partially digested food is pushed forward into the small intestine to begin the process of absorption in the small intestine or elimination through the rectum. The stomach is empty, and the pyloric sphincter closes while the gastroesophogeal sphincter opens to allow the process to start all over again. The system that nature designed is ingenious and simple and works quite well for most of us.

But babies are not most of us. Babies are different. The gastroesophogeal sphincter in young babies is not a fully functional muscle until approximately ten months of age. Instead of opening and closing, the sphincter stays open all the time. Unlike an adult's, when a baby's stomach forcefully contracts to move the partially digested food into the intestinal tract, the churned up food not only pushes forward past the pyloric sphincter, but it also pushes backward through the open esophogeal sphincter. The esophogeal muscle is not ready to do its lifelong task of closing when the stomach contracts. Therefore, food can easily be regurgitated by babies through this open sphincter.

In addition, babies enjoy sucking on a nipple, whether breast or bottle, and sometimes drink more than their small stomachs can handle at any one time. With an open sphincter, a major anatomic obstacle to regurgitation in adults is removed; in babies, the excess breast milk or formula just comes up and out. There is no harm to the baby in this process as long as the baby is retaining enough calories to grow and enough fluid volume to maintain a normal urine flow.

Also, remember that babies are small; the distance between their stomachs and their mouths is only three to four inches. Whereas in adults, the distance is twenty-two inches or more. Again, an anatomic obstacle to regurgitation is removed.

The gastroesophogeal sphincter is not the only immature body part in a baby; in fact, babies have many immature body parts. Picture it this way. Your new baby does not walk even though each baby has two legs and feet with muscles, tendons that attach to the foot bones, and nerves that could direct those muscles to move those feet. And yet your young baby does not walk. Why? Simply put, the musculoskeletal system is immature, and babies need an average of thirteen months before they figure out how to work the muscles, tendons, bones, and nerves work together. Your doctor does not tell you your newborn has a problem because your baby can't walk. No one is prescribing special braces and exercises to get that little guy or gal up and about. No one is developing a treatment plan or new drugs for this "problem."

We have invented the name gastroesophogeal reflux disease (GERD) and have developed treatment plans and new drugs to force that immature gastroesophogeal sphincter to grow up and function before its time. This is a "pediatrick." Nothing is wrong with your baby.

Let's use another analogy to illustrate why nothing is wrong. Your baby has a muscle at the rectum to control his or her bowel movements. This muscle is the rectal sphincter. The rectal sphincter too is immature, and thus, your baby poops randomly and in an uncontrolled manner. It amazes me that no one has decided to call this tension elasticity rectal disorder or TERD and developed medications and diagnostic workups to discover why this muscle is not working. Of course, the workup for TERD would be absurd.

Unfortunately, GERD has been embraced by the medical community. Many babies endure invasive diagnostic workups and are medicated when the poor, unfortunate immature gastroesophogeal sphincter doesn't work as it does in adults.

In 2003, two newborns joined my practice while I was away on vacation. One was bottle-fed, and the other was breast-fed. The bottle-fed baby was taking one and a half ounces of formula per feeding by his second day of life and was often "yucking" it up. While in the hospital nursery, his diet was changed to a soy formula because he was diagnosed with a "milk allergy". This soy formula made no difference. Two days later, when he was still "yucking" up his formula, he was changed to an even further-refined, and more expensive, soy formula. Again, this refined soy formula made no difference. At one week of age, he was continuing to "vomit," so he was put on a totally predigested formula, which is very expensive. His parents were told to keep him in an upright position after feeds. The diagnostic reason given for all these formula changes was that this baby had both gastroesophogeal reflux disease (GERD) and milk allergy. Yet, despite his having two "diseases," he managed to be one full pound above his birth weight at three weeks of age. Such weight gain is excellent in an infant this young.

The second infant was a breast-fed baby who also was diagnosed with a "disease" by one week of age. She was spitting up after every feeding; thus, she was diagnosed with GERD. This baby was put on an antacid to control her regurgitation symptom, and the parents were told to keep her in an upright position for one hour after each feeding. She had regained her birth weight by two weeks of age, a very appropriate weight gain.

Returning from my vacation, I examined these infants. Both infants were obviously thriving, and I relayed this fact to the parents. Understandably, the parents believed that their babies had GERD. They were concerned that their babies suffered discomfort from regurgitating, as adults seem to do. No one had explained to them why spitting up is a normal function for babies. I reviewed with these parents the anatomy and physiology of digestion in a baby.

I advised the parents of the first infant to return to cow's milk formula and of the second infant to return to a regular nursing regimen without medicine. These babies continued to grow and develop normally. They also both continued to be "cheesy" and "yucky." However, now, instead of distress, the parents are happy and relieved that their children do not have diseases. They are saving on the cost of fancy formulas and expensive medicines. The effort of cleaning up a baby and the cost of extra laundry are insignificant compared to the anguish and cost of having a baby with a disease.

More importantly, what was the difference between what my daughter did twenty-nine years ago and what these two babies did in 2003? In fact, there is no difference. All three of these infants had gastroesophogeal reflux, but in 1974, it was not defined as a disease. Gastroesophogeal reflux in babies under ten months of age was not a disease in 1974, and it is not a disease today.

In adults, gastroesophogeal reflux can be a disorder for which there are appropriate treatments and medications. As in so many other ways in our society, we have allowed this disease in adults to "trickle down" and become a disease in infants. We not only encourage our babies and children to grow up more quickly, but we assume that symptoms, which may signal a health problem in adults, may be a health problem for our children as well. While GERD has validity as a disease in an older age group, it has no validity as a disease in infants. The technology exists to document that infants have reflux, but it is inappropriate to apply this technology to babies. Technology confirms what we have always known clinically—that normal infants under ten months of age have reflux. We should not go further—but we do. The popularization of GERD in the media certainly has made it one of the more catchy diagnoses. Unfortunately, once diagnosed, treatments and remedies are soon to follow.

I practice pediatrics in the Boston area, but this rush to diagnose GERD is not limited to Massachusetts. On my vacation in the southern part of the United States, a mother asked me for my opinion about her four-month-old baby. The mom told me that the infant had vomited large amounts of each feeding in the first two weeks of life. This baby's formula had been changed a few times, and now he was being fed the most expensive formula. He was also medicated with an antacid and a hydrogen-ion blocker. He had had an ultrasound and a pH probe to evaluate the anatomy of his gastrointestinal system. Despite these measures, he continued to vomit after meals. Of course, other than his reflux, no anatomical abnormalities had been discovered. Most importantly, this full-cheeked baby with pudgy arms and legs weighed 17.5 pounds at only four months of age. Clearly, he was perfectly normal!

Why, then, do those in the medical profession diagnose him with a disease? Why have physicians and other health-care professionals redefined a normal bodily process into a disease?

The answers are probably a combination of reasons that lie at the roots of our fast-paced society and our current health-care system. These systems have encouraged the redefinition of normal gastroesophogeal reflux into gastroesophogeal reflux disease. GERD is certainly the rave these days. Newspapers, magazines, and websites report about it on otherwise slow news days.

First, making a quick diagnosis is easy and takes no time. Explaining to parents why many babies "yuck" up is a time-consuming event.

Second, in today's medical environment, spending time to explain normal functions to patients is not cost effective and may not be reimbursed by health insurance companies, especially when there is a limit on the number of well-baby visits per year.

Third, our fast-paced society looks for quick answers to deal with a problem. It is not surprising, then, that we are quick relay to parents that their infants have "reflux" or "milk allergy." Saying those words is not time consuming for the physician. Coding a patient visit with a diagnosis is more likely to be reimbursable by insurance. And parents are reassured that the problem is being addressed and treated.

Fourth, today's diagnostic technologies can prove that what my mother called "cheesy" is the refluxing of stomach contents. Having demonstrated by technology that reflux exists in babies, we feel compelled to label it, package it, and sell it. "Cheesy" doesn't sell nearly as well as GERD.

I see and hear about many referrals for GERD of babies who are actually quite healthy and growing normally. These babies throw up their dinners, so they have to endure mega-workups and treatment plans. Some babies even undergo surgery to tighten the sphincter muscle. You are told to change to a soy formula or to begin a prescription antacid to decrease acid secretion. You may be referred to a gastroenterologist who will insert a pH probe or perform an esophogoscopy (a fiber optic tube inserted down to the stomach to observe reflux). You are instructed to feed your baby small amounts frequently and keep him upright for an hour after feeding. Needless to say, by ten months of age the babies are cured,

NOT because of all the interventions and treatments but because they outgrow the symptoms when the sphincter muscle matures.

We must recognize that some symptoms are normal. Rather than devoting time and dollars to treatments and cures, we need to spend time educating parents about this fact. Your grandmother would have said you have a "cheesy" or "yucky" baby and that would have been the end. Today, we say you have a baby with a disease for which there are treatments. And treat this disease we do.

Our health-care system has created an industry focused on this "disease." We have created business for pediatricians and pediatric gastroenterologists who can cure their patients by ten months of age and be reimbursed for their efforts. Pharmaceutical companies have converted the prescription medications for adults into useable strengths and formats for babies, presumably boosting sales. Formula companies have found a new market for their many specialized formulas. Hospital ultrasound and radiology departments are reimbursed well for documenting that gastroesophogeal reflux is present.

Is there any harm in treating GERD with antacids and hydrogen ion-blocking medications? Are there risks involved in pursuing invasive workups? Most medical therapies and diagnostic procedures have potential side effects. Only time will tell if long-term problems will emerge.

Please understand that a rare baby may have a problem called pyloric stenosis. In twenty-seven years of practicing pediatrics with thousands of patients, I have seen only a handful of cases. And babies with pyloric stenosis or any other significant problems related to vomiting and reflux become ill and have decreased urine output. They do not retain enough calories to gain weight. If your baby is vomiting up part of each feeding but is gaining weight, growing on a proper growth curve, and urinating, your baby is normal. If your infant is failing to grow and, more importantly, has a decrease in urine output, then a full evaluation is of course indicated.

Surely, at the very least, these formula changes and medications make parents think that there are real digestive problems in their babies. These false conceptions can last a lifetime and take on a life of their own. Many times, I have heard parents say of their eight- or nine-year-old, "Megan has always had stomach problems." The truth is Megan has never had any stomach or bowel problems other than what the medical community has led her parents to believe.

Rather than attempting to alter our normal human physiology, we should be teaching parents to accept the fact that babies are "cheesy" and "yucky" because they are babies. We know that babies who throw up but grow well are not endangered. In labeling that which is normal as a disorder or disease, we may be putting ourselves and our children in harm's way. So take a little advice from my non-medically trained mother. If your baby is growing well and wetting its diaper on a regular basis, then learn to ignore the recurring nuisance of cleaning up after your baby's "yucking" up. When you were a baby, you probably did the same thing to your mother and baby, look at you now.

Parent Vince C. wrote,

As a new parent, always feel nervous about baby's condition. My kid's story may be just an ordinary story. But an unordinary man took good care of her and her parents. Our little one was vomiting the formula constantly in first week. It made I and my wife extremely uneasy. I called Dr. Heller for emergency assistance. First, it was Nancy answering the phone. I don't know why, I just feel kind of comforted because I sensed something about caring. Then Dr. Heller spoke to me. Based on my description, he diagnosed it was not serious situation and told us observing baby's urine condition and met him next day.

When we met him next day, he quickly examined the little one and verified she is fine. Then he spent a lot time giving us fundamental knowledge of physiology of baby. He draw some graph to demonstrating why baby so easy to vomit.

Not only he took care of baby, but also he "took good care" of parent as well. Because comfortable parent will take good care of child.

And I never forget, he asked us where we are from. When the baby still crying, he comforted baby and said Taiwanese "mon how," which mean don't cry. It concluded a nervous visit a comforting trip.

At the moment I told my wife, Dr. Heller was some guy sent by God to guard the kids.

14

Home Security System Installed Free of Charge

Frequently, when I am confronted with a question for which there is no clear answer, I think about what my caveman ancestors did in a similar situation. What happened when our ancestors became ill? How did they fight off infections, whether viral or bacterial? The primary answer is quite simple; the caveman relied on his immune system.

Full-time Security 24/7 at No Extra Charge

For our local and national security, we have police forces, the FBI, the CIA, and the Dept of Homeland Security. For our bodies, we have an immune system—a fully integrated, intelligence-gathering and deciphering, defense-strategizing organization. For tens of thousands of years, newborn babies have arrived with a fully installed (although not fully functional) immune system. A review of the various integrated components helps us to understand and respect the system's abilities.

Spies, Informants, and Officers on the Beat

The job of our local police forces is to maintain order in our communities. In addition, the FBI, CIA, and Homeland Security rely on spies, informants, street agents, and electronic surveillance to gather intelligence about enemies or threats to our national security. This information is usually sent to a local base or headquarters for interpretation. The immune system is able to perform these same functions.

The immune system has two divisions: the natural or innate immune system, which, like police officers on patrol, reacts immediately to new crises; and the acquired immune system, which responds to detailed information about an enemy to form a response, but which takes time to make this response. Both arms of the immune system are important to maintain well-being.

On the intelligence-gathering and detection side, almost any particles that enter your child's body through the openings of the nose and mouth or through breaks in the skin are immediately intercepted by cells called macrophages. These cells provide continuous surveillance for foreign materials. The macrophages travel throughout the body using the arteries, capillaries, and veins as their highways to access and monitor every corner of the human body. They also visit lymph nodes regularly. After encountering any unusual material or chemical structure, as, for example, a virus, a bacterium, or an allergen, the macrophages engulf the foreign material and deliver it to the regional lymph nodes. The macrophage cells are like spies or informants who get some information and transmit it to headquarters where the information is processed. The regional lymph nodes function as headquarters and are a hub of activity in the overall system.

Refer All Suspicious Characters to Regional Headquarters, the Lymph Nodes

Lymph nodes, found behind the ears, in the neck, under the arms, in the groin, at the elbows and knees, and within the chest, throat, and abdomen, are local interrogation centers. Some of the more famous lymph nodes are the adenoids and tonsils in the neck region. Usually found just under the skin, the lymph nodes feel like small round smooth movable bumps and are often mistakenly called glands. They work continuously and usually do not cause much attention or alarm. However, when fully engaged in a protective battle, they become more noticeable. In full battle mode, as an important line of defense within the immune system, lymph nodes are tender, swollen, and working their hardest to overcome the enemy invader by instituting defensive measures.

The lymph nodes serve three primary roles. First, they devour locally what they can of the foreign object and attempt to destroy it. Second, they study the invader and analyze, classify, and store information about it. Third, they begin the process of manufacturing antibodies to ward off the attack. The lymph nodes may be tender and painful when performing these functions, but they are working for the defense of the entire body.

Reports and Sightings Sent to Central Command

Information from the lymph nodes is transmitted to more central locations in the body over a system of vessels or tubes called the lymphatic system. Basically, the enemy invader is brought to a central interrogation unit, where the foreign object is examined and a defense strategy is devised. White blood cells bring the invader to the local lymph nodes where the counterattack is planned. The immune system needs about seven days to two weeks to examine the foreign material and find a weak point in the enemy. During this process and immediately afterward, the immune system begins a specific counterattack by manufacturing specific antibodies that can attach to and immobilize that specific invader. Over time, this amazing immune system creates antibodies for every foreign matter that enters the body. Not only does the immune system make specific antibodies, but quite remarkably, it stores that information, in many cases, for the entire lifetime of that individual. This is recognized as "a state of immunity." If the same invader ever attacks again, the strengthened immune system no longer needs a seven- to fourteen-day delay to respond. With a second assault, antibodies are immediately released to protect the body. This is why, as immune parents, we are not at risk to reacquire chickenpox if our children develop the disease.

Alarm Systems and Warning Lights

Additionally, the body's immune system comes equipped with two major alarms that send signals to the body that all is not well. The first alarm is the activity that occurs in the lymph nodes themselves, and the second is the system's ability to generate fever.

The Mission of the Lymph Nodes: To Protect and Capture

As noted above, the lymph nodes become tender and swollen in response to an attack. The regional lymph nodes that are closest to the site of infection are the first to respond by becoming enlarged. Locally, in the case of a break in the skin, white blood cells migrate through the capillaries to the site of injury and engulf bacteria. The accumulated white blood cells (granulocytes) are recognized as pus, providing an immediate attempt to localize an infection. Deeper infections of soft tissues, as in the mouth or throat, for example, will result in swollen tonsils at the back of the throat and swollen lymph nodes, "glands," in the neck. While sore throats and swollen lymph nodes may be uncomfortable, they are part of the normal immune response; as such, they are part of the solution to the infection rather than part of the problem. Too often, doctors and patients rush to remove tonsils and adenoids because they frequently become swollen and uncomfortable rather than understand that those parts of the immune system are accomplishing important tasks. Chronically enlarged tonsils, which block the upper airway, should be evaluated and, in rare cases, may need to be removed. My view is that we should hardly ever remove these or other parts of the immune system. Indeed, all lymph nodes work throughout your life. They defend against outside and inside enemies.

The Enemy Without: Infectious Agents and Allergens

Lymph nodes are there to protect and defend you against infection and invasions from the outside world. Polio, for example, is a viral illness that can cause muscle weakness and paralysis. Spinal poliomyelitis causes paralysis only in the legs. Bulbar poliomyelitis affects not only leg muscles but also the muscles of respiration. Those with bulbar polio require "iron lung" machines to keep them alive. Why do some people develop only spinal polio while others developed the far more life-threatening bulbar poliomyelitis?

Fifty years ago, the *Journal of Pediatrics* published a study of the polio epidemic. That study revealed a critical fact: those who had undergone tonsillectomy were three to four times more likely to contract bulbar polio, thus suffering from respiratory failure. The authors speculated that the absence of tonsils and adenoids decreased the effectiveness of the immune system. Apparently, those lymph nodes had a local protective influence in preventing the polio virus from compromising the respiratory nerves that stimulate the respiratory muscles.

The immune system also offers protection from allergies. Allergens, like pollen and animal dander, are foreign proteins and chemical structures that enter our bodies and trigger an adverse reaction by the immune system. Lymph nodes have the ability to create various types of antibodies. Some of these antibodies not only attack and dispose of the foreign material, but may also trigger other responses, including skin rashes or respiratory wheezing. The confusing and complex story of allergies will be discussed in a separate chapter.

The Enemy Within: Cancers

Another function of the lymph nodes is to capture and interrogate suspicious cells that might arise within the body itself. These abnormal cells are called neoplasms or cancers. We have evidence that the immune system monitors our bodies for aging cells and abnormal cells that might become cancerous or dangerous.

Not only does it perform a monitoring function, but it also has the ability to destroy these cells. Patients whose immune systems are weakened by medication given after organ transplantation to prevent rejection have an increased risk of developing cancers. The immune system is obviously not perfect in its role as a cancer detector or fighter. We have a lot more to learn about its role in these processes at the present time.

Fever: The Unsung Hero

The occurrence of a fever is the second major component of the alarm system. Like swollen lymph nodes, fever is a friend, not an enemy. The same white blood cells and macrophages, which first begin to repel an invasion, also send a signal to the brain to crank up the thermostat of the body. Chemicals called endogenous pyrogens cause the central regulatory area of the brain to increase the body temperature. While you may think, "Oh my goodness, my baby has a fever, and that's bad," the immune system of the individual with the fever views it as a critical aid in fighting the infection.

Fever not only signals the invader's presence, but it also contributes to the counterattack by the body. Since fever causes an increase in the heart rate, more blood gets pumped around the body, and consequently, more infection-fighting white blood cells are being dispersed through the system.

Fever to the Rescue by Making Porous Walls

In addition, fever is associated with an increase in the permeability of the capillary walls. Capillaries are the smallest-sized blood vessels in your body and are in direct contact with all muscles, organs, tissues, and skin. This close contact permits the exchange of oxygen, carbon dioxide, nutrients, and waste products. During times of fever, various chemicals are released that increase capillary permeability and chemotaxis (see below). An increase in capillary permeability means that larger white blood cells and greater numbers of white blood cells can leave the vascular system and move toward the site of infection in the soft tissues of the body. Chemotaxis refers to the ability of these cells to travel through the soft tissues to the infection. In essence, infection-fighting white blood cells are better able to leave the capillaries and enter the tissues of your body that are under attack. The migration of white blood cells is enhanced during fever, and the result benefits the immune system.

Fever: Your Body's Warning Light

An auto's "engine warning signal" can indicate a problem with the temperature, oil level, or compression in the engine. A mechanic needs to examine the engine before a serious problem ensues. Fever is like an "engine warning light" and can be due to different causes. Simple problems like over-clothing or an over-heated room may cause an infant's fever. Fevers can occur in a child who is dehydrated and merely needs more fluid. Fever may also signify the occurrence of an infection due to a virus, bacterium, or inflammatory condition.

In sum, fever is a warning that the immune system is fighting an infection or responding to other inflammatory conditions. Parents should check with their pediatrician who is able to sort through the many causes of a fever and whose response will depend on the exact age of your baby, as well as other signs and symptoms. Fever in and of itself is not specific to a certain condition.

The Immune System Is Impressive

Basically, your new baby comes fully equipped with a built-in security system that is almost matchless in its performance abilities. The immune system recognizes foreign bodies and foreign agents and categorizes them into either infectious agents, allergenic agents, or nonspecific inflammatory agents. Unlike most security systems, it not only detects a problem and sends out an alarm, but it is also able to respond independently to the crisis at hand. Without intervention on your part or that of modern medicine, it uses countermeasures to repel the attack and guards against future assaults of the same kind.

Too Good to Be True: Fully Installed but Delayed in Functioning

By this point, you must be saying to yourself, "This security system is almost too good to be true." Your skepticism is quite correct. The immune system's features are installed, but those features are not all fully functional on the first day of life. In fact, if you read the fine print in your newborn owner's manual, you will realize that the immune system needs a full year to develop before all its amazing features can run at reasonably full efficiency. During the first three months especially, the system is immature and often non-responsive or inadequately responsive to certain pathogens.

Maternal Antibodies to the Rescue

Fortunately, nature is aware of this lack of efficiency of the immune system in the first year and covers most of the potential risks. At the moment of birth, a baby is preloaded with antibodies that are actually those of the mother. Since the circulations of the mother and fetus lie side by side in the placenta, antibodies from the mother are passively transferred to baby late in pregnancy. For this reason, extremely premature infants are even more susceptible to infection than full-term babies.

Not all antibodies are able to cross the placenta, but a significant number of maternal antibodies are transferred. Some acquired by the infant are short-lived and disappear by two to three months of age. Others remain in the baby and provide protection for up to a year or longer.

You may wonder, for example, why we wait to immunize children for chickenpox until a year of age or why we delay immunization for measles, mumps, and rubella until fifteen months of age. The answer is that if the mother had had these diseases or had been immunized against them, she will transfer protective levels of these antibodies to the fetus. If we try to immunize a child for these illnesses too early, the maternal antibodies still present in the baby may influence the proper immune response of the infant, preventing the infant from acquiring an appropriate level of immunity.

But Maternal Antibodies May Not Be Sufficient

A serious problem arises if the baby is attacked by an agent for which there is no passively transmitted maternal antibody; in that case, the infant may be in a helpless situation. Since the baby has no maternal antibody protection and is unable to manufacture his own quick response, infecting virus or bacteria may have an advantage. This unique set of circumstances dictates that any baby who develops a fever in the first three months of life must be seen and fully evaluated by a medical care provider.

Full evaluations of infant fever are no fun for parents or babies. Depending on the history and physical findings, a full assessment may involve needle sticks for blood tests, bladder catheterizations for urine examinations, spinal taps, and chest x-rays. Are these tests necessary? Absolutely, and your baby's life may depend upon such measures. Some very rapidly progressing and devastating illnesses can occur during these first twelve weeks. On more than one occasion, I have seen a perfectly normal baby succumb to a group B streptococcal infection in less than a day. I have seen infants become very dehydrated and toxic due to urine infection. While admittedly these cases are rare, the consequences of failing to administer early treatment are unacceptable.

Fever under twelve weeks is a warning sign that cannot be ignored. After three months, the newborn's immune systems begin to function more like adults and the response to fever becomes a bit more measured. Nevertheless, parents are encouraged to contact their baby's medical care provider when a fever develops.

Detective Work: Finding the Bad Apples

When I teach Harvard medical students both in the hospital and in the office setting, I explain to them that of our many roles as physicians, the one that is challenged almost daily is that of being a detective. A good detective learns to identify the criminal or the enemy using a technique called profiling. In medicine, we use a form of profiling. The family or last name we generally give to all our adversaries is "ITIS." The very large ITIS family has only bad apples. Among its members are the familiar Tonsil Itis, Pharyng Itis, Mening Itis, Ot Itis, Bronch Itis, Nephr Itis, and Arthr Itis, just to name a few. How do we recognize members of this group? We look for four distinguishing characteristics. In medical school, we are taught the Latin names, which have a poetically unifying sound: Rubor, Tumor, Calor, and Dolor. In English, these words are translated as redness, swelling, fever, and pain, all of which are clues generated by the immune system.

- **Redness** at the site of an infection as a consequence of the inflammatory response is a reflection of increased blood flow and the migration of anti-inflammatory cells to the site of irritation.

- **Swelling** is also generated by the immune system. The regional lymph nodes enlarge, and white blood cells and plasma accumulate at the site of the viral or bacterial infection, causing swelling.

- **Fever** develops as a part of the overall immune response due to bacterial breakdown products and chemical signals released by immune cells.

- **Pain** results from the swelling and inflammation. An infant signals the existence of pain in a nonspecific way by crying or acting as if he is "just not himself" or "is unable to get comfortable." An older child can verbalize.

Both doctors and patients can be detectives; discovering an ITIS is not difficult if one pays attention to the clues that the immune system sends out.

For eons, this system had single-handedly kept our species alive and evolving. We began this chapter with the question, "How did our caveman ancestors handle infections?" Clearly, our immune system has kept our species alive, but the system isn't perfect. Can we improve on it so that fewer people succumb to diseases or injuries?

The First Improvement by Ancient Ancestors

Yes, people have been able to improve on the immune system as installed by the manufacturer. Thousands of years ago, our predecessors made the first improvement. When our children were young, we traveled to visit Grandma Rose in Texas. Taking a slight detour to the Dallas/Fort Worth area before making our way to Galveston, we visited a museum in Fort Worth that has a marvelous exhibit about prehistoric people. Amidst the display was the skull of a cave person who had had a hole drilled through his parietal bone. The healing at the edge of his bone provided clear evidence that the "patient" survived the procedure and lived for several years beyond that moment of drilling.

We can only guess at the reason the hole was made: Was it made to drain blood that may have developed from head trauma? Or was it made to drain the pus of an infection? Pus is a combination of white blood cells and bacterial debris. Drainage of pus from a wound accelerates the healing process and usually produces a successful result. This technique was used by our ancient ancestors; the Greeks called this "laudable pus." Later, during the Middle Ages, "barbers" drained wounds and abscesses. For centuries, people have boosted the success of the immune system by the simple addition of drainage.

Immunizations—Not Very Modern at All

The next and quite stunning improvement has its roots in 1022 AD when, according to written accounts, a Buddhist nun ground up the scabs of smallpox victims into a powder. She then blew this powdery substance into the noses of nonimmune people. This practice, known as variolation, was an attempt to give someone a mild form of the disease, hopefully sparing that person from the more severe ravages of smallpox. With some success, variolation continued over several hundred years. Epidemiologists have estimated that this practice decreased the total number of fatalities from smallpox by tenfold.

A mere 774 years later, in 1796, Dr. Edward Jenner developed a vaccine against smallpox. He had noted some similarities between cowpox, a cattle disease, and human smallpox and realized that milkmaids rarely died during epidemics of smallpox. He extracted fluid from a cowpox pustule and inoculated a boy. Eight weeks later, Dr. Jenner exposed the boy to smallpox; the child did not contract the disease. This was the first successful vaccination against an illness that had, at that time, a 30 percent mortality rate.

In 1980, almost two hundreds years later, the World Health Organization declared that the entire world was free from smallpox. A terribly disfiguring and frequently lethal disease had been eradicated by an immunization program. During the last century, many vaccines against both viruses and bacteria have been developed. As with the story of smallpox, many children today do not suffer physical and mental disorders or death because of these vaccines.

Improvements by Modern Society: Antibiotics

The fight against bacterial diseases received another powerful weapon in 1928 when Sir Alexander Fleming accidentally noticed that a mold called penicillium could destroy certain bacteria. In 1940, Drs. Howard Florey and Ernst Chain isolated the active ingredient, now called penicillin, and that step led to its use as an antibiotic to fight infections. During World War II, penicillin was responsible for saving the lives of many soldiers who suffered from wound infections. As an aside, penicillin saved the lives of many Spanish bullfighters, whose deep wound infections were treated successfully with penicillin. Spaniards were so grateful that a statue honoring Dr. Fleming was erected in Madrid's bullring.

Since the discovery of penicillin, scores of new antibiotics have been developed. The immune system alone could not conquer all bacterial infections. The combined effort of the immune system and antibiotics has protected millions of lives from death or damage that bacterial diseases can cause.

While antibiotics and immunizations provide major enhancements to the immune system, we should always remember that the immune system on its own has single-handedly protected our species for thousands of years. Still, antibiotics and immunizations are magnificent allies and are welcome additions in the fight against infectious diseases.

Parent Louis M. wrote,

My favorite story about Dr. Dan occurred when he was confronted with the collective energies of my parents and my mother-in-law. They demanded to know why my almost 2 year old daughter had some routine malady.

"Because she is a member of the human race," he told them.

Parent Christine H. wrote,

Several years ago I visited Boston with Michael and our second son, John. John had experienced continuous ear infections for 5 months. Even though Dr. Heller was no longer our pediatrician because we had moved to another state, he was still kind enough to take my call and advise me regarding John's ear infections. He explained to me that many doctors are over-diagnosing ear infections and that if John has no fever then he probably has no serious infection.

Talking to Dr. Heller put me at ease (and rightly so). After that John had no more ear infections.

15

Boosts for the Immune System

Immunizations and Antibiotics at Extra Cost: A Reasonable Option

The development of immunizations and the discovery of antibiotics changed the course of human lives dramatically. The immune system has protected us from diseases for thousands of years. Our ancestors realized that drainage of pus, hot compresses, and some herbal remedies could help fight viruses and bacteria, but the immune system did lose some battles. Deadly enemy invaders like smallpox and polio viruses and invasive bacteria could leave us crippled, mentally damaged, or dead. While there have been many discoveries about how human bodies work and new technologies to diagnose and treat illnesses, none has affected more lives than immunizations and antibiotics.

Rounding on Interesting Cases

An important part of the training of new physicians and nurse-practitioners is to visit in-hospital patients regularly. In medical jargon, this process is called rounding or making rounds. Whether thirty years ago or today, medical trainees are encouraged to make rounds on patients and to visit especially those with "interesting" diseases. In fact, the very rare and unusual cases are actually presented to the entire staff at hospital grand rounds. The concept is that medical trainees who are exposed to these cases will be able to recognize those same diseases after training is completed, and trainees become fully practicing physicians.

Where Have All the Diseases Gone? Long Time Passing

As a pediatrician, I am relieved that many of the diseases that afflicted children thirty years ago have been eradicated in modern societies. As a teacher, I feel satisfied that I can no longer show my students some of those "interesting" cases. Young doctors and nurse-practitioners rarely see kids with measles, mumps, or rubella. Hospital wards are no longer filled with polio victims who need iron lungs to breathe for them. Gone are the emergency room visits of children with Hemophilus influenza epiglottitis (the epiglottis is a flap of tissue protecting the upper airway) or blue-domed facial cellulitis (an inflammation of soft tissue of the face), both of which are potentially lethal infections. Vaccinated children no longer suffer extensive neurologic damage from chickenpox or measles encephalitis (an inflammation of the brain). In much of the world, mumps no longer causes the sterility of boys, and rubella no longer threatens fetuses, whose rubella-infected brains were subject to microcephaly (impaired growth and development) and subsequent mental retardation.

Immunizations have had a wonderfully dramatic effect on the lives of children and their families. And yet some parents do not want to immunize their children.

A Matter of Luck?

Some parents argue that because of wide-spread immunization, their children are not at risk. They feel lucky and reason that "If everyone else is immunized, then my children are not at risk," a concept known as herd immunity. Do not rely on the immunization status of others to protect your child from vaccine-preventable diseases. Our planet has become rather small with the advent of modern air travel. Exposure to illnesses from areas beyond one's neighborhood is now commonplace. Recently, the SARS virus spread from continent to continent in a matter of days.

What will happen when your un-immunized child becomes a world traveler as an adult? Staying at home does not offer protection, and exposure to infections here or abroad is definitely out of parental control.

Some parents are fearful of immunizations because of reports of autism occurring after certain vaccines. In 1998, in the British journal *Lancet*, a report was published that the measles, mumps, and rubella combined vaccine (MMR) was related to the subsequent development of autism. Every major scientific review of this topic had demonstrated that autism is *not* related to MMR immunization. In 2004, authors of the *Lancet* article wrote to the *Lancet* to "retract an interpretation" that autism and inflammatory bowel disease were related to the MMR vaccine. Dr. Simon Murch said, "There is now unequivocal evidence that MMR is not a risk factor for autism—this statement is not spin or medical conspiracy but reflects an unprecedented volume of medical study on a worldwide basis."

Extensive Evidence Exists that Our Vaccines Are Safe

I am quite sure our vaccines are safe. Current monitoring and scrutiny by local, state, and federal agencies and current research about vaccines ensure their efficacy and safety. For example, some people wondered if the mercury-containing preservative thimerisol might be related to autism, a neurodevelopmental disorder that affects communication, social, and reasoning skills. A Danish study covering a seven-year period reviewed the records of 537,303 children. This study demonstrated no difference in autism rates between vaccinated and unvaccinated children. Similarly, extensive research has shown no link of the MMR vaccine to autism. In any case, the Food and Drug Administration has established new guidelines that have virtually eliminated thimerisol from childhood vaccines.

Sadly, we do not know the cause of the rise of autism in our children. Many researchers are examining various possibilities to determine what causes a condition that is affecting an increasing number of children. The focus on finding the cause of autism is reasonable, even compelling. And it is equally reasonable, even compelling, to acquit those suspects that have been proven to be not guilty.

Reassuringly, our government and health-care systems have mechanisms in place to respond to concerns about our vaccinations. Several years ago, a new vaccine against rotavirus was released. Rotavirus is a common cause of diarrhea in infants and young children and, in some cases, leads to dehydration and death. The rotavirus vaccine had the potential to reduce not only the discomfort of the diarrhea, but also the need for hospitalization of infants and children with this illness. Soon after the vaccine was approved, a few dozen cases of intussusception were reported. Intussusception is a condition where the intestine slides into itself causing severe pain and risking the loss of blood flow to the intestine. Intussusception can be a life-threatening condition. The response of governmental agencies and vaccine manufacturers was rapid and definitive. The vaccine was withdrawn immediately and has never been reintroduced. In this instance, the evidence supported a finding of guilty as charged. A new rotavirus vaccine is being developed, which is not associated with an increased risk of intussusception.

The Centers for Disease Control (CDC), the American Academy of Pediatrics, and the Advisory Committee on Immunization Practices (ACIP) all study and evaluate the efficacy of vaccines. All vaccines currently in use are safe and effective and have been proven over time to be without significant side effects.

Decision Making 101

I spend most of my day helping people make decisions. For every decision we make, I know there was a decision we rejected. We reach that fork in the road so well described by Robert Frost. In medicine, as in many professions and businesses, much of our decision making is based on a benefit-risk analysis. In other words, we examine the benefits and risks of doing X as well as the benefits and risks of not doing X.

Equate X with immunizations for this illustration.

- Benefits of immunizations—excellent protection against debilitating and life-threatening diseases

- Risks of immunizations—minor reactions of fever, soreness, and the remote possibility of, as yet unsubstantiated, long-term sequelae

- Benefits of no immunizations—no concerns about possible, unsubstantiated sequelae of the vaccines

- Risks of no immunizations—the likelihood of severe illness from debilitating and life-threatening diseases

Any realistic look at immunizations will come to the conclusion that the diseases that the vaccines protect against have far worse consequences than the side effects of the vaccines themselves.

Not a Matter of Luck, Be Smart

Many of today's grandparents know someone whose life was affected by polio, diphtheria, pertussis, tetanus, measles, mumps, rubella, hepatitis, meningitis, or chickenpox. Today's parents, however, hardly know anyone who had these dreaded diseases. The difference in the experiences is totally due to immunizations.

While I was training to become a doctor, I saw illnesses I will never forget. I saw perfectly normal children with measles that had spread to their brains. The resulting inflammation of the brain tissue, called measles encephalitis, led to significant neurologic breakdown; these children were left with shattered bodies and minds. I saw kids with severe chickenpox; they developed encephalitis and never again had normal thought processes. When on rotation at Cambridge City Hospital, I worked on a ward with kids who choked and gagged on their mucous secretions from pertussis (whooping cough).

As eleven-year-olds, Roger, Eric, Peter, Russell, Jay, and I always hung out together after school to play stickball. Then, Peter's brother, David, contracted polio. We never played with Peter again. Our parents would not allow contact with him; all we knew was that polio was a very frightening disease. We thought that Peter's brother, David, had the plague. Peter had to wear a mask over his mouth in school. Peter and David and their parents eventually moved to another town.

Nancy's Story—Polio Wrecks Havoc on Families

My father, Dr. Martin Schneider, radiologist and pioneer in the field of radiation oncology, was in the intellectual and physical prime of his life in 1948. He had returned to Galveston, Texas, from service in the U.S. Army only three years before and was director of the Radiation Therapy Department at the University of Texas Medical Branch at Galveston. In May 1948, he was thirty-five years old when a polio epidemic struck the Texas Gulf Coast. As a physician, my dad was working tirelessly to provide care for polio victims when he was infected with polio. He was immediately hospitalized and confined to an iron lung, which is a machine that breathes for those who cannot breathe for themselves.

Why did polio strike my dad? He was an adult at that time, and polio was primarily a disease of childhood. Was he so tired and worn down from long hours at work that his immune system was weakened? Was there a link between my father's tonsillectomy when he was a child and the bulbar polio he contracted when he was thirty-five? We will never know for certain why that virus chose my dad. But what we do know is that polio does wreck havoc on its victim and his or her family.

Cooped up in that iron lung day after day, my father wondered each day if it would be his last. He could hear and speak, but he couldn't breathe on his own, much less move his arms, legs, or any other part of his body. My mother spent her days, and many nights too, at the hospital, helping to care for my father, reading to him, and talking with him to keep his spirits up. After a few months in the hospital, my father was able to breathe on his own again, and he and my mother traveled to Warm Springs, Georgia, for physical therapy and recuperation. My father never regained the use of his legs and was confined to a wheelchair for the remainder of his life. Still in his intellectual prime, he died at age fifty-three from respiratory failure because his diaphragmatic muscles, ravaged by his polio, finally gave out.

Our family was profoundly affected by polio. My dad was very ill and then very dis-
abled before his early death. During the acute phase of polio and afterward, my mom
shouldered much of the responsibility for caring and supporting our family. My dad
required assistance from us all in most aspects of everyday life, from dressing in the
morning to getting in or out of the car or having his wheelchair pushed wherever we
went. He couldn't do what most fathers could like play baseball or lift us in the air or
ride with us on roller-coasters. He was often tired and would even fall asleep at the
dinner table during family conversations. In countless ways, some small but others all
too large, his disability and early death changed my family's functioning.

Luckily for our family, my parents had wonderful friends who were willing to care for
my siblings and me while our mother ministered to my father at the hospital. I was
only three years old at the time, and my brother was a baby. My sister, however, was
nine years old, and as soon as the word spread among the parents of her peers that our
father had been stricken with polio, none of her friends were allowed to play or be
with her.

My sister was devastated. Terrified that our father would die, she wasn't even allowed
the comfort or companionship of her friends to help her cope with our situation. As she
became more agitated and upset, the only solution that our parents could think of to
ease her distress was to send her to live for some time with an aunt and uncle in the
northeast. My sister never forgot her rejection and loss.

Hemophilus Influenza B Attacks the Brain

About twenty years ago, the totally normal and lovely little two-year-old boy of
my friends died of meningitis. His brain was attacked by bacteria called *Hemophi-*
lus influenzae B (HIB). Another child, a patient of mine, survived the brain
inflammation from this bacterium, but the inflammation destroyed her auditory
nerves; she is totally deaf. This bacterium can also inflame the epiglottis (a flap of
cartilage which folds over the top of the trachea or upper airway), causing life-
threatening respiratory failure. Today, because of the HIB vaccine, this lethal
bacterium has been banned from doing its dirty work. Most newly trained pediatricians have never seen a case of invasive HIB disease.

What Would the Victims of These Preventable Diseases Want?

Most children abhor shots and cry when receiving vaccinations. Some parents
don't want their children to receive vaccinations because of the fleeting pain from
needles. But the children with measles encephalitis or chickenpox encephalitis

can't abhor or think about anything because they are dead or profoundly retarded. The children who suffered from Hemophilus influenzae type B meningitis can't hear their own cries or those of others because they are deaf or dead. Polio victims and their families would rather have a quick moment of discomfort rather than die, be significantly disabled, or be forced to uproot their lives. Those with pertussis cannot speak when they are choking and gagging on their secretions.

Needless to say, I do not have much patience for those who want to deny their children the safety provided by immunizations. I don't feel badly about giving immunizations because I understand the significant benefits. I know the anguish of the families and children who have had these preventable diseases, and I know that their suffering is far greater than the anguish of the shot. I know I am doing children a great service by immunizing them.

Antibiotics: The Immune System's Second-greatest Assistant

Unfortunately, researchers have not yet developed immunizations against every disease; and occasionally, foreign invaders, in the form of both bacteria and viruses, can overcome the immune system, and the system fails. At other times, the immune system just doesn't respond quickly enough to fight off an infection, or it seems weakened or debilitated. The responsiveness of the immune system is affected by licit and illicit drugs, by our mental states and sense of well-being, and by viral infections. While it is well-known that the AIDS virus suppresses the immune system and leads to significant opportunistic infections, other virus can have a similar effect to a much lesser degree.

In 1928, with the discovery of penicillium by Dr. Fleming, the immune system gained a worthy assistant and a tremendous boost in its defense of the body against bacterial infections. By 1940, the antibiotic penicillin was being produced and being followed on a growing scale by many other antibiotics. The age of "wonder drugs" had begun. In partnership with the immune system, antibiotics have shortened the time to recover from bacterial infections, thereby reducing the chance that the immune system's slow response would permit it to be overwhelmed by a foreign agent. Since antibiotics begin to work immediately, they truly appeared as "wondrous."

Just Like Superman, WONDER DRUGS Have Limitations

As helpful as they are, antibiotics, however, cannot replace the immune system. Donata, a patient of mine years ago, had aplastic anemia, a condition in which one's bone marrows does not make any new red or white blood cells. Without white blood cells, Donata was at such high risk of infection that she lived in a hospital in a special tent and had no contact with the outside world. Despite such extreme precautions, she developed an infection in her bloodstream called bacteremia. She was treated with high doses of antibiotics intravenously for over three weeks, and yet every single day bacteria were cultured from her blood. I was amazed that, despite the antibiotics, bacteria were still free to roam through her body. Her immune system was ineffective, and antibiotics alone could not save her. I felt so frustrated when she died. We had done all we could with our "wonder drugs," but she needed a working immune system to aid in the fight against her infection.

Baby Boy O'Leary was born at the old Boston Lying-In Hospital on Longwood Avenue. I had just begun my private practice career and felt comfortable with my medical abilities and the armamentarium of drugs I had at my disposal. Baby Boy O'Leary was a full-term baby, delivered vaginally without any complications.

But Baby Boy O'Leary was born in 1977. At that time, a vaginal culture of the mother was not routine. Today, such a culture is performed routinely to identify bacteria called group B streptococcus, a cousin of the common group A streptococcus that causes sore throats. If the mother is positive for group B strep, she is either pretreated or the baby is evaluated with laboratory tests to determine if he is infected. However, in 1975, we did not understand that babies born vaginally were at risk from group B strep if their mothers carried this bacterium.

Shortly after his birth, Baby Boy O'Leary began having breathing difficulty. As part of our immediate and full assessment, we drew blood for a blood culture, and the baby was treated with high-dose antibiotic therapy in the event that an infection was causing his difficulties. Twenty-four hours later, Baby Boy O'Leary was dead, and the cultures of the blood showed group B strep. Again, the "wonder drugs" had failed. The baby's immune system was not yet fully functional, and antibiotics alone cannot always win the war. Today, because of our awareness of the severity of this infection, pregnant women are screened for this condition and treated prenatally if necessary. Keep in mind two important points. First, antibiotics are an adjunct to a working immune system. Second, antibiotics can't compete against viruses.

Extra! Extra! Read All about It: Virus Beats Wonder Drug

Viruses and bacteria are not at all alike and are treated differently by the immune system. Different types of white blood cells are sent out to immobilize and destroy bacteria and viruses. At any given moment, blood contains white blood cells called granulocytes that deal with bacteria and white blood cells called lymphocytes that deal with viruses. Basically, the two infecting organisms are so different that the immune system needs two different defense mechanisms. Antibiotics aid granulocytes in fighting off bacterial invaders. But antibiotics offer no help to the lymphocytes that fight viruses.

Whenever a child spikes a fever, 85 percent of the time the cause is due to a virus. Yet, perhaps 60 percent of the time, doctors will prescribe an antibiotic.

Asking Too Much of Our Superheroes

Understandably, doctors and parents want our superhero wonder drug to come to the rescue whenever an infection sickens a child. However, since antibiotics are completely ineffective against viruses, it is not surprising that wonder drug fails when deployed to treat a virus. An antibiotic is not needed because, 85 percent of the time, illnesses are due to viruses.

Wonder drug is not always necessary, even against bacterial infections. For instance, otitis media (middle ear infection), of which 50 percent are due to viruses, does not require immediate antibiotic treatment in children who are over two and half years of age. The reason for this is that most ear infections, even those due to bacteria, will drain and resolve on their own without treatment once the patient is older than thirty months. Thus, the best practice is to wait a day or two to see if the ear infection resolves itself without antibiotic intervention.

Sore throats are common and may be caused by viruses or bacteria, but the only sore throat that needs antibiotics immediately are those due to group A streptococcus. We actually treat strep throat to prevent acute rheumatic fever and possible rheumatic heart disease rather than to make your child's throat feel better. The use of antibiotics is unnecessary for viral illnesses and is not always necessary for all bacterial infections. Remember, the immune system has put up quite a respectable defense for thousands of years before wonder drug appeared on the scene.

Part of the problem in antibiotic overuse is that pediatricians all too often think that parents will be unhappy if their child is not treated with medicines. Often, I spend more time explaining why I won't treat an infant or child with antibiotics than I would spend if I gave in and provided a prescription to ensure a "happy customer." However, the issue is not about having happy customers. The American Academy of Pediatrics has organized a nationwide campaign to educate parents and physicians about the overuse of antibiotics and to encourage them to use antibiotics less often than we currently do.

Extra! Extra! Read All about It: Bacteria Beat Wonder Drug

Overuse of antibiotics actually contributes to a major problem called antibiotic resistance. Just as the body responds when it is attacked by an infectious agent, so too the infectious agent retaliates if attacked. Bacteria are equipped with defense mechanisms to alter either their own structure or the structure of the antibiotic. The more those bacteria are exposed to a given antibiotic, the more adept they become at developing resistance to that antibiotic. As antibiotic resistance increases, we are forced to develop newer and stronger antibiotics. This approach, however, has its limitations. We may encounter a time when we will not be able to outsmart bacteria with newer and stronger antibiotics. We would not need newer antibiotics if there were less antibiotic resistance. There would be less antibiotic resistance if antibiotics were used appropriately. Our general overuse of antibiotics is aiding and abetting the enemy. Wonder drug needs a break.

Back to Decision Making 101

At any office visit, you and your pediatrician have to work together to decide what is best to do for your child. The pediatrician-parent relationship needs to be based on trust and honesty. The first concern has to be the health and safety of the child; making parents happy has to take a backseat. Antibiotics are not always the answer.

So What Did He Say About Immune Systems, Immunizations, and Antibiotics?

- Babies have an immune system that is quite incredible and works round the clock to protect and defend them.

- Immunizations are a must and an adjunct to the baby's immune system.

- Antibiotics are superheroes, and like all superheroes, they have some weaknesses.

- When it comes to antibiotics, one has to choose when to use them correctly, which one to use, and learn not to abuse and overuse.

Parent Patricia L.: Dr. Heller Appreciated the Involved and Informed Parent

Charlie received his polio vaccinations before the days of orally administered vaccines, so he had all the shots. When we were coming up on the time for the first vaccines for our second son, Patrick, Dr. Heller gave us a brochure that explained the new oral vaccines. After reading the brochure, my husband and I decided that even though it meant a few shots for Patrick, we did not think that the benefits of the new vaccine outweighed the risk that it might not be as effective and we just felt uncomfortable because the oral vaccine included live virus, albeit weak.

When my boys and I arrived for the wellness visit, I told Dr. Heller our decision. He said, "You want me to give him a shot?"
I replied, "Yes, we read that brochure."
Well, you'd have thought I said the Magic Words. "You read the brochure? You read the brochure?" he exclaimed.
"Yes," I said. He said, "Come with me, come with me, come with me," and then he grabbed me by the hand and took me down the hall to Dr. Bunnell: "This lady read the brochure!! Amazing!! She wants the kid to have a shot. Somebody read the brochure!" When we left Dr. Bunnell, we ran into Betsy (the head receptionist) and Dr. Heller told her all about it too. I never imagined that reading a brochure could make anyone so happy!

16

Two-month Visit: Prepare for Big Changes, Both Inside and Out

Among the most noteworthy developments at eight to twelve weeks of age is the maturation of the nervous system and the beginning of coordinated muscular movements. As noted earlier, the respiratory, cardiac, and endocrine systems assumed basic functions very shortly after birth. Excretory functions of the kidneys and bowels were in place from the first day. By two months, every parent would had changed enough diapers to verify that statement. The gastrointestinal system was in working order by the end of the first week and capable of digesting and absorbing food. The increase in length and weight of the baby confirms that those systems are working. While several bodily systems become fully functional shortly after birth, the nervous system in humans requires significant time to mature. Unlike most mammalian babies, who walk in the first week of life, human babies need twelve to eighteen months to accomplish this task. While it may take us longer to accomplish many of the gross motor tasks that other mammals achieve earlier, we surpass all other mammals in our fine motor, language, and personal-social skills. In the end, we outsmart all other mammals.

Two Nervous Systems for the Price of One

A baby is born with more than one nervous system, the peripheral nervous system and the central nervous system The peripheral nervous system connects the brain to all muscles. Both systems, under baby's control, are responsible for gross and fine motor movements. The nerve endings in the muscles have the ability to release chemicals called neurotransmitters that excite or inhibit contractions of the muscles. A great deal of fine-tuning is necessary to release just the right amount and type of neurotransmitters to obtain a coordinated movement of the muscle.

Embedded in the peripheral nervous system is the autonomic system. These autonomic nerves are controlled by a structure deep in the brain, the hypothalamus, and together they are responsible for blood pressure, temperature regulation, and a number of other automatic functions. The hypothalamus is also the main center for regulating hunger and for stimulating the endocrine organs to secrete their hormones. Through this mechanism and other related ones, sexual development is therefore dependent on the hypothalamus.

The central nervous system or brain holds court inside the skull. At the base of the brain is the brain stem. The brain stem is responsible for heart rate and for breathing without thinking. All of this happens without one's direct control, and these functions occur on an involuntary basis.

The medulla, the lowest part of the brainstem, contains monitoring sensors for oxygen, carbon dioxide, acid, and blood pressure levels. It reads these signals and responds by sending out messages to the lungs and heart to increase or decrease their rates to maintain balance. The medulla takes over in the first few minutes after a baby is born. It continues to mature over time and becomes better at making the appropriate adjustments to regulate cardio-respiratory stability and temperature control.

Above and behind the brain stem is the cerebellum. The cerebellum is responsible for coordinating the muscles and maintaining body equilibrium. In humans, the cerebellum is functional but very immature at birth. In mammals that walk in the first week, the cerebellum is more developed than in human babies. All mammals come equipped with the basic brain stem and cerebellum. Humans are special in how much more brain tissue is enclosed in our skulls.

Atop the cerebellum is the cerebrum, and these two big lobes are the image that most people have of the brain. This amazing organ maintains links to all parts of the body to deal with and respond to pain, hunger, thirst, and environmental stimuli such as sight, smell, sound, touch, and taste. Over time, the cerebrum regulates sleep, though it never sleeps. Above all else, it has the incredible ability to think, to imagine, and to remember. The brain is often thought of as a living computer. That analogy is not true and, in many ways, does not give justice to the uniqueness of the human brain. A newborn's brain has distinct areas dedicated to certain skills. One area is for language, one for motor skills, one for memory, and a unique area to integrate learning. The ability to integrate information and learn skills is the feature that takes the longest to mature and to function at the high levels humans are able to attain. This complex organ system needs considerable time to become fully functional.

One of the most fun and exciting things about being a parent or a pediatrician is to watch that neurological development. Right before our eyes, we can see the subtle signs that the brain is actually developing. A major part of each well-child visit is to look for those subtle changes and enjoy the progression of achievements that come one little step at a time.

The First Time Ever I Saw Your Face

For example, at the two-month visit, a baby begins to have conjugate gaze. This means that both eyes begin to work together, and the infant can fix on and follow an object. When that object is a parental face, the baby has provided a thrilling moment. Parents know the joy of finally seeing their baby make eye contact that is not merely random movement. While it may not seem like much of an achievement, it is a colossal step forward. Prior to establishing conjugate gaze, each side of the brain was working independently. Conjugate gaze demonstrates that the brain is beginning to operate as a single unit. Also, prior to the development of conjugate gaze, a baby knows his mother by her touch and smell. Now, due to his brain's development, the baby can put a "face" on the mother he only knew by feel and smell.

As this ability to focus and follow objects improves over time, a baby will be able to use his vision to reach out and touch a specific object. But at this stage, arm and hand movements are still not well coordinated. Basically, the ability to fix and follow with the eyes is the first step in the development of hand-eye coordination. The infant brain is beginning to observe and store information that will eventually lead to the development of fine motor movements that surpass those of any other mammal on earth.

Juice and Tummy Time

At two months old, babies enjoy some juices between regular bottle and/or breast-feedings. I recommend that parents dilute juices with water to decrease the sugar load. Dads enjoy feeding babies too, and juice bottles provide another opportunity for a father to nurture his baby.

All babies need time on their tummies to begin using muscles of the upper torso as well as to practice lifting their heads. An interesting consequence of the national "back to sleep" program is that babies have poorer head control and delayed ability to roll over. They also can develop significant flattening of the back of the skull. On the other hand, they do reach and grab things earlier since their arms are free to make these maneuvers. Thus, babies benefit from both positions, and it is reasonable to give your baby equal time on his stomach and on his back when he is awake.

Also, babies at this age need to exercise their leg muscles. Allowing them to push off with their feet and support some weight is a perfectly fine way to exercise their legs.

Sunrise, Sunset

New biologic rhythms are beginning to be established by two months of age. In the uterus, the sun never rises or sets, and the placenta never rests in its job to provide nutrition and remove wastes from the fetus. After delivery, a baby first begins to experience the changes in light associated with the changes from day to night and back again. But these environmental changes in light will not be part of a baby's biologic clock for at least two to three months. The rise and fall of the sun enable the brain to establish biologic rhythms over time. These biologic rhythms can be measured. Body chemicals of melatonin, serotonin, and steroids have rhythmic blood levels over the course of a day. Sleep, like fixing one's gaze or grabbing, is a slowly learned skill, first requiring the establishment of these biologic rhythms.

Under twelve to sixteen weeks of age, we should not expect a baby to sleep through the night. Reasonable demands for comfort and nutrition from birth to four months are the responsibility of parents and should be met. Many parents find these issues to be challenging but also very rewarding. Caring for a baby is an important part of the bonding process and the establishment of a long-term relationship. But notice the word *reasonable*. If an infant is demanding to nurse every minute, that demand is unreasonable. If an infant is demanding to be held every minute, that demand is also unreasonable. Even at this early age, limit setting is an important part of parenting.

Rarely does a baby become a good sleeper before three months of age. The best advice for parents is to brace yourselves; know that sleep deprivation is coming, and grab naps whenever you can. I remember being awakened when our daughter was six weeks of age, not by her crying (which I was used to), but rather by Nancy's crying out, "What do you want?" At this time, Nancy had not had more than three hours of sleep at one stretch for six weeks, and she was really sleep deprived and miserable. I took our daughter and told my wife to go to bed. Somehow, I felt I could settle Marissa down. What did I know? I was only a pediatrician. Within thirty minutes, I too was crying out, "What do you want?"

Two years later, while on vacation in St. Thomas, I held our six-week-old son, Matthew, on a porch facing the Caribbean moon at three o'clock in the morning. Speaking toward heaven, I asked if any West Indian god would like a miserable child. I still did not understand at that point in my life that none of us controls another person's sleep.

In retrospect, I think that our constant holding, rocking, burping, and passing off of our children from one to the other became a source of constant stimulation and agitation for our babies. A child behaviorist, Dr. Peter Gorski, brought this to my attention years later, and what follows is the gist of his position about sleep in infants.

Don't Over-stimulate

Think about whatever you do for a living. You have a job with a certain number of tasks and a time period to perform these tasks. One day, your supervisor says, "We have a problem." A co-worker is sick, and your assignment is to complete your work and your co-worker's tasks for the day. You buckle down and realize this will be a rough day, but you can do it. Five minutes later, the supervisor returns and tells you, "We have another problem." The child of another co-worker is sick; that colleague won't be in, and now you are required to complete his work as well. Soon, you throw your head back and scream and cry because the boss has just overwhelmed your ability to handle the extra work.

Now think about your baby, who has a very immature nervous system. The slightest touch, noise, and movement can elicit a full Moro or "startle" reflex. This is a primitive reflex in which hands and legs fly outward and the infant cries. This reflex probably served a very useful protective function when the cave woman mother left her baby while she was hunting or foraging. The slightest touch, noise, or movement of a predator could trigger the startle reflex; suddenly, the cave baby no longer appears to be a harmless, motionless object but a much larger-appearing, noisy danger. Perhaps this reflex helped to scare off predators who might otherwise have fancied that newborn as lunch. Whatever the evolutionary significance, this reflex disappears when the infant is ten to twelve months of age (and able to swat at a predator).

Today's babies receive many stimuli. Much of it is educational for babies and fun for parents. But at times, multi-stimuli represents nervous system overload. We hold and burp our babies—stimulation number one. We rock back and forth—stimulation number two. We pass our infants from caregiver to caregiver—stimulation number three. We sing and place our babies in swings—stimulation number four and five. We have done all we can to comfort our babies. But by now, any baby's immature nervous system is so overloaded that it is in a constant state of "startle" reflex. While our intentions have been to calm our babies down, we have only revved them up. The crying intensifies; we can't see that we caused our babies to cry louder and harder.

The best action is to swaddle babies and lay them down, thereby allowing them to have less rather than more stimulation. Will parents still hear cries for thirty minutes to an hour? Definitely. We need to allow infants a respite from dealing with the extra unintentional stimulations that are not helping, but are intensifying the situation. We also need to understand that babies will learn to organize themselves and to figure out how to fall asleep by theirselves.

Nancy's Story: What a Difference a Third Child Makes

As a new mom, I thought that the best way to put our daughter to sleep was to trick her by letting her fall asleep before placing her in her crib. We had a routine. I changed her diaper and dressed her in nightclothes. I made sure that her door was closed; no household noises or pets could disturb our tranquility. I sat in the rocking chair in her darkened room. While I rocked her, she nursed. When she stopped sucking for at least ten minutes, I knew that she was asleep. I carefully rose and walked gingerly to her crib, taking care not to jolt or awaken her. When lowering her into her crib, I prayed that she would not wake up and begin to cry. If she did, we began the rocking-and-nursing ritual over again. If she didn't, I was pleased and tiptoed as I left her room, quietly closing the door behind me.

The initial phase of the ritual was very rewarding for me; I enjoyed the hour of peace, tranquility, and bonding with my baby. Even after the second round, I still felt satisfied. Beyond that, my patience gave out, and I would feel frustrated and aggravated that I was spending so much time, as many as two or three hours, putting my baby to sleep. Luckily for me, she was willing to be tricked most of the time.

As I became a more experienced parent, I had an entirely different experience with our youngest child, Sara. When putting her to sleep, I didn't worry so much about household noises. By then, we had two older children who were not going to tiptoe around the house while their baby sister slept, so worrying about this issue would only have put me in direct conflict with them. And in reality, their noisy antics did not wake her. I did rock and nurse her too and was grateful when we could bond without interruption from a well-meaning sibling.

But the biggest difference in my approach was to place her into her crib when she was still awake or wake her gently and then put her into her crib. In this way, she learned easily and with relatively little anguish on my part that she was responsible for falling asleep. On rare occasion, she would cry herself to sleep, probably releasing some pent up frustrations known only to her. But I would never categorize her sleeping habits as problems or concerns because I had learned how to help her learn to sleep.

When to Intervene

With babies, nothing succeeds like success. If your baby is sleeping well and you hold, rock, burp, and pass her around, then you can ignore all the above information. However, if your baby is driving you to tears over her failure to sleep and her lack of sleep is preventing you from your sleep, understand that you can take positive steps to change the situation. You may be over-stimulating your infant. Give your baby and yourself a respite. Let her cry after you have ensured that she is sated, dry, and doesn't have a fever. Help her learn that she can fall asleep on her own.

Like many issues in pediatrics, infant sleep issues are within our control only to the extent that we can set the stage for sleep. For example, we can prepare babies for bed by changing clothes and diapers, we can offer a breast or bottle, and we can lay them down in their cribs. But we cannot force them to close their eyes; we do not have control over that most important factor of sleep. Our anxiety and frustration may relate to our lack of control. Obviously, no one wants a parent-infant relationship filled with anger and frustration.

Let Me Whisper in Your Ear

Besides the improvement in coordinating vision at two months, babies demonstrate the first subtle signs of language. Babies begin to coo. Unlike the crying and shrieking sounds made to signal general discomfort, cooing is a soft vocalizing noise made in the mouth and is pleasing to the ear. As all parents do, we loved it when our babies began to coo. Before there was any cooing, babies' only vocalization is to complain. Cooing is a sound that says, "Thank you, Mom, you are doing a good job." Cooing is also the sound that indicates to a pediatrician that the rudiments of language are becoming organized.

Two Months: You've Come a Long Way, Baby

- Gross Motor: When lying on his stomach, a baby can raise and turn her head from side to side. She will also push off when held in an upright position and bear some weight.

- Personal-social: Your baby will begin to regard your face, and sleep will be improving. If sleep is a problem, take steps to change the situation. Teach your baby that she can fall asleep on her own; over-stimulation of an infant's nervous system contributes to sleep problems.

- Language: Cooing represents a major step forward.

- Fine Motor: Visual coordination is being fine-tuned, but fine motor skills are not evident yet.

Dr. Heller's Common Sense Advice to a New Mom: Parent Patricia L.

Once, when Charlie was an infant, I put him on the bed and turned away to get something. Next I knew he was lying on the rug on the floor.

Panicked, I called Centre Pediatrics and Dr. Heller took my call. He asked me some questions, and then told me I could bring Charlie down for a look-see if it would make the new Mom more comfortable. I did. After looking him over, and assuring me that Charlie was not scarred for life, his advice was: "Always put the baby on the floor; he cannot fall off the floor." Brilliant!

"Take them out in the rain. Babies can get wet. Water won't hurt them."

"Forget about the infant bike seat. What if you are out riding on the road and something hits you, even if the baby is safe which chances are he will be, should you get hurt, now there is a baby who can't speak for himself and you are off in an ambulance."

17

What's for Dinner?

Among the many roles I play as a pediatrician, teaching medical students and residents is one of the most fun and challenging. I have had students from Boston medical schools such as Harvard, Boston University, New England Medical Center, and some from as far away as Pittsburg. Whether these students are with me for one session or for weeks or months, I want them to learn certain basic principles.

Principle number one: Ask questions and reach conclusions.

Principle number two: Wonder what would happen if the truth was just the opposite of your conclusions.

This past year I began to ask my students what they knew about solid feedings for infants. I was surprised to learn that little class time was spent on this subject. When should we start to feed a baby? What should we start with and how much? We reviewed much literature and contacted several experts in the field. We discovered that there are many opinions but very little science. In fact, every grandmother, parent magazine, nutritionist, and primary care provider has a distinct opinion on this topic.

Let's look at the whys and wherefores of current feeding practices in America. Despite my training in a very good hospital, I was not well prepared in giving practical advice to patients about a myriad of day-to-day simple topics, including advice about nutrition. I listened to my elders and assumed what they said had some basis in fact. Over the years, I came to realize that most of our advice was truly "off the cuff" if not "off the wall."

Feeding Babies Is as Simple as Pie If You Start in '75: Bring It on at Six Weeks

In the early 1970s, the rules were very clear. First, we fed a baby when he was six weeks old. This was a radical change from the advice given in the fifties and sixties. During that earlier period, babies were fed beginning at two weeks of age. By the seventies, the American Academy of Pediatrics had decided that two weeks was much too soon to feed a baby. Pediatricians feared that babies might choke or gag if fed solids at two weeks of age, and thus, solid feeding was delayed until six weeks of age.

Second, the rule about what to feed was also clear. Even when babies were fed at two weeks old, a certain protocol for the introduction of foods had been worked out. No change was made in that general protocol. Babies were fed rice cereal twice a day. The cereal could be mixed with formula, breast milk, or water, and the amount was two to four tablespoons. Babies ate this same regimen for a week before parents introduced the next food to be sure that there was no change in bowel habits or any rash suggesting a food allergy. Usually, "orange" or "yellow" vegetables followed rice cereal. These included squash, carrots, and sweet potatoes. Again, babies ate "orange" or "yellow" vegetables and rice cereal for one week. Next, parents introduced applesauce and banana. At this point, the baby was over two months old, and parents introduced "green" vegetables as well as the P foods—peaches, plums, and prunes. At three months of age, the baby had yogurts and meats.

The No-no's in the 1970s

Just as there were rules about what foods to offer babies, rules about what not to offer were clear and definitive. Rule number one: Do not give a baby any honey for two years due to the chance of botulism poisoning. Rule number two: Do not give chocolate, nut products, or strawberries until nine months of age because of the increased likelihood of allergies if these are given early. Rule number three: Do not give eggs until six months of age for the same allergy issues. (As a side note, some pediatricians advised to give either the whites or the yolks at four months. I could never remember which part was permissible and felt it was too difficult to totally separate those two parts of an egg, so I just told parents to wait until six months of age.)

Until six months of age, all baby foods were to be a custard consistency. At six months of age, foods could be of a more solid consistency; and by one year, babies could be on ordinary table food, except for obvious foods like nuts and raisins that could cause choking.

Oh, Goodness! We Got It All Wrong: It Should Be Three Months

Within a year of my beginning the fine art of private practice, the American Academy of Pediatrics decided to change the rules. Various committees reviewed the feeding advice that American families were being given. Many specialists, including allergists, immunologists, gastroenterologists, and nutritionists, expressed concern about foods and the timing of their introduction. Breast-feeding advocates questioned whether foods might affect the protective antibodies in breast milk. The major change that occurred was that the introduction of solid foods was delayed until three months of age.

Babies no longer were fed at six weeks of age. As to which foods to give, the rules remained unchanged. The sequence of rice cereal, "orange" and "yellow" vegetables, apple, banana, "green" vegetables, meats, and yogurt was left untouched. As before, foods needed to be a custard consistency until six months, and then more solid consistencies could be given.

Oh, Goodness! We Got It All Wrong Again: It Should Be Six Months

In 1981, the American Academy of Pediatrics again decided that its advice of a few years before was incorrect. The academy recommended a further delay in the introduction of solid foods until six months of age. I had been in practice for six years and had seen three major changes in the recommendations as to when to start feeding babies.

One of the driving factors in the 1981 change related to the increasing rate of allergies in infants and children to various foods. A consequence of normal growth is that the walls of the intestines become thicker and more mature over time. The assumption was made that a thinner bowel wall would be more likely to pass a foreign protein into the body than a thicker, more mature bowel wall. Basically, medical scientists postulated that the thicker bowel wall of a six-month-old would be more protective against foreign proteins entering the body, and thus, we might be able to decrease the chance of allergic reactions. As before, the question on what to feed babies did not change. The sequence of rice cereal, orange vegetables, apple, banana, green vegetables, meats, and yogurts was left untouched. Of course, what did change dramatically was the delay of eight or nine months in the introduction of foods with greater solid consistency.

Oh, Goodness! You've Got to Be Kidding; We Have Gotten It All Wrong Again!

More than twenty years later, the facts are very clear. We now have more reported food allergies, nut allergies and asthma, than ever before. Evidence is mounting that allergies and asthma in children increase when exposure to allergens occurs later in life. In other words, when infants and children are exposed earlier to potential allergens, those infants and children appear to be less likely to develop allergies and asthma. The concept that the thickness of the bowel wall was the important factor did not pan out to be true. It is somewhat ironic that our advice to delay food introduction to an older age may have contributed to rather than decreased the problem of allergies.

When it comes to food, the opposite of what we thought might be true has come up over and over. I have sat behind my desk and told people to use margarine rather than butter only to see that advice reversed. Currently, we are moving away from the low-fat, high-carbohydrate diets that the food pyramid glorified for so many years.

Delaying the introduction of solid foods until six months may also be in the category of good in theory but not in practice. In my practice, I have returned to a recommendation of three to four months as a safe and reasonable time to introduce solids. Babies' swallowing mechanisms and protective gag reflexes are mature by this age. We know from the history of feeding that even most six-week-olds were able to chow down solid foods of custard consistency.

So What Shall We Feed Them?

The next question is what foods to introduce first. Before answering that question, we need to return to principle one—question the source of the information and the evidence for the information. Why did the sequence of introducing rice cereal, followed by orange vegetables, apples, bananas, and green vegetables, and ending with meats and yogurt originate fifty years ago? The answer is simple: diarrhea.

Diarrhea and Infant Feeding: You've Got to Be Kidding

From the beginning of recorded history, diarrhea has been the leading cause of death in infants and children all over the planet Earth. Even today, dehydration and shock secondary to diarrhea claim more lives worldwide than any other illness. Along with vomiting, diarrhea causes so much concern because of the possible consequences to the health of the child. Diarrhea with vomiting and fever keeps pediatricians' phones ringing and emergency rooms busy.

What does that have to do with feeding a newborn baby solid foods? When pediatricians sat down to design a diet for a two-week-old baby, they wanted to be sure that their diet did not cause or exacerbate diarrhea. We all know that some foods tend to bind up one's bowels and some foods cause a looser bowel consistency. Peaches, plums, raisins, prunes, and green vegetables belong to the latter group. If baby's first foods were among that group, parents would notice loose stool, usually when it got out of the diaper and went down the leg in no time. Immediately, parents and pediatricians alike would wonder whether this diarrhea was due to an infectious agent or a consequence of the loosening foods. Thus, the decision to avoid stool-loosening foods as a baby's first introduction to solids was an easy one and did not require deep thought.

On the other hand, rice, carrot, squash, sweet potato, and banana have the marvelous ability to turn stools into bricks. All of these foods are constipating. No in-depth research was done when we chose the classic sequence of constipating foods. Nor did we change the sequence when we began feeding children at older and older ages. From a pediatrician's point of view, the phone call about a baby who had not pooped for five days is much easier to respond to than the phone call about a baby who had had five loose stools in one day. For the first situation, we can suggest the introduction of some peaches, plums, prunes, and green vegetables; for the latter situation, we have to wonder whether the stools are loose as a result of dietary intake of loosening foods or whether this child has a bowel infection.

What about Allergies and Delaying Chocolate, Nuts, Eggs, and Strawberries?

During my training, I neglected to ask why we had some foods on our no-no list. I was told or assumed, based on common knowledge, that the introduction of eggs before six months and chocolate, nuts, or strawberries before one year could cause a baby to become allergic. I mistakenly accepted this on faith. And for years, I gave this advice to my patients.

Fortunately, my patient population is multicultural and multiethnic. Over the years, I have asked parents from different parts of the world what they introduce for their babies' first foods and what foods they avoid. The answers are fun on one level and informative on another level. Obviously, all foods do not exist in all places on this earth. And clearly, human beings have babies and live in all parts of the earth for thousands of years. That different cultures and different geographic areas have unique feeding protocols should not be surprising. What is surprising is that we seem to believe, in America, that we have the right answer.

In India, the initial food seems to vary depending on the region of the country. In some parts of that country, the first food is a bean or lentil paste, and in other parts, the first food is a millet grain crushed into a paste. In India, the only food not given to a child under one year old is wheat. In Vietnam, the first food is a mixture of red and green beans and rice that is stir-fried and made into a paste or custard. Peanut oils and peanut products are not avoided in the cooking and preparation of this food. In parts of the former Soviet Union, yogurt is the first food. Among some Muslims, the first food is a date; their newborns are given a tiny taste of date at birth. This is the earliest solid feeding that I have heard of in my questioning.

At last count, all these infants seem to be surviving and doing well on very different diets with very different rules. You should be beginning to think that there are many rules, but perhaps none of them makes much sense. And indeed you are quite correct. There should be no rules on what food to begin feeding to babies.

Oh, Goodness! There Are No Rules

In 2002, the American Academy of Pediatrics published its updated nutrition handbook.

It's over five hundred pages long and quite heavy. *What* food should we start first? I searched through the handbook to find the current recommended sequence of foods. There is no recommended sequence. The Nutrition Committee of the American Academy of Pediatrics does not exist in a vacuum. Policy statements are affected by political and economic issues. The United Nations and World Health Organization have committees that deal with children's needs. While listing a sequence of foods could be a fine approach, committee members had to consider the consequences of selecting specific foods that might not be available throughout the world. "Regarding the question of which foods to introduce and in what order, the answer should be whichever foods you choose and whatever order you choose."

When should we start feeding a baby solid foods? The handbook is very noncommittal on this topic. Apparently the Breast-feeding Committee of the academy suggests that we should encourage no solids at all until six months of age. Many breast-feeding advocates believe that the only nourishment a baby needs is breast milk.

The Nutrition Committee on the other hand is concerned that breast milk is lacking in zinc, iron, and vitamin C and that earlier solid food introduction at three months makes good sense. How could breast milk be lacking in these nutrients? Haven't our babies been feeding on breast milk without a problem for ten thousand years? This is an interesting question. Clearly, the diet of humans on earth for the first ten thousand years was much different from that which lactating mothers eat today. At its simplest, people ate more dirt with their meals thousands of years ago. And the diet of our ancestors was much higher in protein and fat and much lower in carbohydrates than is our diet today. Breast milk content is, to a certain degree, dependent on the mother's diet. Most likely, breast milk today is not quite what it used to be and may lack in certain minerals. So the handbook gives a wide range in timing about when to begin feeding. A tongue-in-cheek answer to the question of when to begin feeding is whenever.

Honey There Is One Rule: No Honey

Just say no to *honey*. The problem is that bacteria can survive in raw honey. Those bacteria can produce a toxin called Botulinum toxin. Botulinum toxin is a neurotoxin that can be fatal to an infant or child up to the age of two. While many advise you to avoid giving honey until one year of age, a safer choice is to wait for two years.

What about Allergies?

On the topic of food allergies, most of us are confused about what makes the most sense. Part of the problem is the over-diagnosis of food allergies. All too often, a facial rash or change in bowel habits or irritable behavior is ascribed to an allergy. Most of these minor problems are not caused by food allergies. If you rubbed your breakfast, lunch, and dinner on your face, your face might also break out with a rash.

Some allergies are true allergies. On the broad picture, some evidence suggests that earlier exposure to allergens leads to fewer allergies and asthma. In light of these findings, introducing foods of all types earlier rather than later makes more sense. Many avenues of research about the increase in allergies are being explored, such as issues of cross-sensitization with baby lotions or soy formulas. But we do not yet have good answers at this time. Some allergies seem to be sporadic in their occurrence and of no known cause. The best advice is not to be concerned about food allergies unless there is a well-documented history of that allergy in the parents or a sibling.

What's for Dinner?

I have a much easier job today teaching a young doctor or nurse-practitioner the correct advice to give new parents about solid food feeding. Begin feeding at three or four months of age. If you are Chinese, feed your infant Chinese food; if Japanese, Japanese food; or any other food you might like. Begin with soft mushy consistency and feel comfortable that by six months the texture can be more solid. Your cave woman ancestor prepared food for her baby by chewing whatever she could find depending on where she was on the planet. The consistency was determined by how long she chewed the food. She then spit out a portion of that chewed food to give to her baby. The bottom line is eat and enjoy.

Solid Feeding

- No honey for two years.

- Three to four months is a reasonable time to begin.

- Pick any menu and see how it goes. The baby will likely decide what he likes and dislikes.

Parent Linda Y. wrote:

Food was an important office visit topic. When we put Mike on solid food, Dan asked what we were giving him beside cereal and baby food. Proudly we answered, "Tofu."

"Poor kid!" was the reply and that's when the photos of children with chicken wings came out. Dinners definitely got more interesting!

Parent Cris O. wrote,

I was concerned that my son was still on the bottle. Dr. Heller said, "Have you ever seen a grown man walking down the street with a baby bottle? DON'T WORRY."

When I was concerned about my son not eating meat, Dr. Heller said, "Elephants are huge and they don't eat meat."

Dr. Heller had a way about him that was off the wall and quirky but we loved that about him.

Parent Courtney H. wrote,

When my mother-in-law worried me that my son wasn't old enough to eat real food—should still be on baby food—Dr. Dan showed me pictures of six-month-old babies from all over the world eating among other things: a sheep's head and sushi!

Parent Katherine D. wrote,

When my daughter was 7 weeks old (she was a big baby), I started her on cereal. AUGH!!! was the reaction of most parents but Dr. Heller didn't flinch when I told him at her 2 month checkup.

Parent Christine H. wrote,

When Michael turned 6 months old Dr. Heller told us he could eat all foods except chocolate, nuts, strawberries, eggs (and no honey until 1 year old). He then proceeded to show us pictures of similarly aged children eating everything from huge drumsticks to pasta to beef etc. Those pictures brought the message home.

18

To Sleep, Perchance to Dream

One of the most exciting things about four-month-old babies is that they finally look like the beautiful babies we have always had images of in our mind's eye. They have "baby soft" skin and are well filled out. Their eyes are wide open, and they smile. They sleep "like a baby" and coo contentedly. But remember that these baby characteristics don't appear until approximately four months old.

Nancy and I fully expected that we would have such a baby from birth. Our expectations were wrong. None of our children had attained that perfection of skin softness and beauty until they were about four months old. The interim weeks were filled with funny facial rashes and acne. With our second and third children, we had accepted the fact that our babies would have many dermatological imperfections. With our first, I wish we had known that babies younger than four months have a face only a parent or grandparent could love.

Another important fact about four-month-old babies is that they are finally capable of a through-the-night sleep pattern, which they develop usually between ten and sixteen weeks old. As mentioned before, neurological development is a slow process. The ability to cope with multiple sensory inputs is not present in the first weeks of life. Sleep patterns too are not fully established before a ten- to sixteen-week timeframe. For exhausted parents, the sad reality is that a baby needs time to learn to sleep "through the night" and to comfort herself. The good news is that by four months of age, she has the ability to sleep "through the night" and to comfort herself.

Who Should Count the Sheep?

When I was a budding nephrology fellow, I gave a postgraduate lecture to 350 physicians. The topic was urinary tract infections in infants and children. I was nervous and hardly had slept the night before. After a brief introduction, the lights in the auditorium were dimmed, and my first of thirty slides appeared on the screen. Within five minutes, I suspected that at least 70 percent of the audience was fast asleep. At end of the forty-five-minute lecture, when the lights came back on, clearly 90 percent of the audience had nodded off. My ability to teach might still have been in question, but there was no doubt about my ability to put doctors to sleep.

That night, Nancy and I spent another fitful night trying to put our three-month-old son to sleep. I could not reconcile how successful I was during the day with putting physicians to sleep but what a failure I was putting my own child to sleep. Later, I realized the misconception of my thinking: I had no control over the sleep of others, including my own children. What do we know about sleep?

The Science of Infant Sleep

Dr. T. Berry Brazelton, the noted child development specialist, studied sleep and crying behavior of infants and children. He videotaped newborn babies and quantified hours of crying and hours of sleep for infants at different ages. He found that in the first week of life, newborns sleep as much as 70 percent of the time and cry very little. Subsequently, hours of sleep decline rapidly so that by two to three weeks of age, babies are awake 50 percent of the time and feeding about every three hours. During wakeful periods, crying time increases at an exponential rate so that between three and eight weeks, babies cry as many as three hours out of each twenty-four-hour period. This crying is not evenly distributed over the hours but tends to come in bouts, especially in the evenings. Not until ten to twelve weeks old is an infant capable of establishing a sleep pattern that includes a seven- to eight-hour stretch at night.

Other studies have quantified chemically and physiologically when a child can establish a normal diurnal (i.e., day and night) sleep pattern. Dr. Stephen Reppert and Dr. Scott Rivkees have made the study of circadian rhythms (daily life cycles) their life's work. Certain chemicals, whose output is regulated by the brain, have peaks and troughs that relate to sleeping. These chemicals include our excretion of endogenous (meaning, made within our bodies) steroids, serotonin, and melatonin. The fact that a day-night-patterned release of these chemicals occurs by ten to twelve weeks is strong evidence that a baby's brain distinguishes day from night at that early age. These findings correlate with the observational studies of Dr. Brazelton.

Finally, researchers have studied infant electroencephalograms or brain wave activity and can distinguish between periods when brains are awake or asleep.

Again, these studies show that by ten or twelve weeks, the human brain can distinguish patterns of day and night, or diurnal pattern. Thus, clinical, chemical, and brain activity studies confirm that by ten to twelve weeks of age a baby has sufficient neurological maturity to differentiate night from day and can sleep up to seven or eight straight hours.

Nancy's Story: I can't sleep; I'm hungry.

Since Matt was our second child, we fully expected that he would sleep through the night by two months old. That is what had happened with our first child. Why should our second one be any different? As our expectations and hopes for a solid night's sleep for ourselves were dashed, we learned the most important lesson of parenting: Every child is different, with different needs and different personalities, even as very young infants.

While Marissa had slept "through the night" (six or seven hours at a time) at only two months old, Matt liked catnaps; his sleep pattern was three hours at a stretch, and then he woke for a nursing session. In fact, by sixteen weeks old, he was awake much of the time and needed to nurse more often. I was dragging myself out of bed in the middle of the night to nurse Matt at least once, if not twice. Frankly, I was exhausted. I could barely keep my eyes open at work, and I had little or no energy for our two-year-old. I understood why sleep deprivation is such an effective torture technique!

At that time, Dan had just begun his practice; and while he knew a great deal about childhood diseases, he had not had experience in common, garden-variety pediatric problems. In desperation, I sought the advice of Albert Cohen, our pediatrician, who was the elder statesman of the practice. His immediate words were "Matthew is hungry. Feed him some solid foods."

I was stunned. On a breast milk diet, Matt had been growing at a very steady clip, and his weight was actually at the upper limits for his height on the growth chart. He had pudgy cheeks and baby fat thighs. How could he be hungry? Besides, we were following the best pediatric advice at that time: breast-feed and delay solid foods until six months. But I was so eager to have a decent night's sleep again that I would do almost anything to make it happen.

Dr. Cohen's advice worked like a charm. Beginning in the evenings, we fed Matt rice cereal and applesauce, which were thought to be the most appropriate foods; and with bulk in his stomach, he finally began to sleep for six to seven hours at a stretch. What a relief! Dan and I both learned from this experience. I learned not to be a purist—the rule about not feeding solid food until six months doesn't work for every baby. Dan focused on the question of why feeding solids helps a baby sleep.

Solid Foods Do Help Babies Sleep

Solid foods have fewer calories than breast milk or formula. Breast milk has twenty-four calories per ounce, and formula has twenty calories per ounce, while cereal, vegetables, and fruits have respectively nine, fourteen, and seventeen calories per ounce. The reason that some babies sleep better when solid foods have been introduced is related to the bulk of solids. Liquid food, despite its higher caloric content, is digested more quickly than solids and, thus, disappears from the gastrointestinal tract more rapidly. Solid food, on the other hand, remains in the stomach and intestines longer than liquid. Thus, the baby feels sated for a longer period of time.

Also, babies are beginning to grow more slowly. Whether breast-fed or bottle-fed, whether eating solids or only liquids, babies do not require the same frequency of feeding as they did when they were younger. Since their growth has slowed, their nutritional needs are also beginning to slow down, thus allowing for less frequent feedings. Both neurologically and metabolically, a four-month-old baby can sleep at night for eight or nine hours at a stretch.

What about Babies Who Don't Cooperate?

We all know babies who don't fit the typical four-month-old model. Parents of a poor sleeper are rapidly losing their wits. They look bedraggled and unhappy. They are semiserious when they joke about offering their baby for adoption. But pediatric book publishers are absolutely delighted at the prospect of sleep-deprived and depressed parents because desperate parents will buy books devoted completely to "sleep disorders" of babies. Hospitals have sleep disorder clinics to address this problem. The medical community has turned sleep into a business. Doctors use billing codes of "disorders of sleep initiation" and "disorders of sleep maintenance" and are reimbursed for their sleep advice and services. Are there really sleep disorders, or is this another pediatrick?

Infant Sleep: Is It Disordered?

Despite all the writings and discussions about this subject, a four-month-old who is not sleeping does not have a disorder. Simply put, that baby has not yet learned how to put herself to sleep. When parents of a four-month-old baby tell me that their child is not sleeping at night, those parents are usually feeling frustrated. I focus on the mental state of the parents and what they have done to encourage their infant to sleep at night.

The most important point for parents to understand is **parents do not control their baby's sleep.** Yes, parents control the time of day that they put their baby in her crib, and they control their baby's environment. They control whether her diaper is dry and whether her stomach is satisfied. They control whether she is warm and whether she is wearing comfortable clothing. But they cannot make her close her eyes and fall asleep. What parents have to do is give their baby the chance to learn how to sleep.

The Answer to the Question, "My baby won't sleep. What can I do?"

Babies integrate new information every day in a neurologic interaction that we call learning. If a four-month-old is still not sleeping at night, the time has come to let her learn how to sleep. Think of sleeping as an acquired skill. I can teach my daughter all I know about hitting a baseball. I can instruct her to watch the ball, keep the bat off her shoulder, and time her swing. We can talk about hitting baseballs during dinner or on our way to little league tryouts. While these steps are part of the process of inputting information into her brain, she has to step up to the plate at some point. She most likely won't hit a home run, much less the ball, during her first time at the bat. In order to become a hitter, she must learn how to put together her vision with her muscle reactions.

In similar fashion, a baby would have to learn how to sleep. The initial input has been her exposure to sunlight, which has helped establish her day and night biologic cycles. Her neurologic system has matured sufficiently as reflected in patterned electrical and chemical activity generated by her brain. She had parental coaching over the first four months, which includes holding, hugging, feeding, and helping her prepare for sleep. Now is the time for her to step up to the plate or, in this situation, lie down in her crib and figure out how to perform this sleep skill herself.

Will our little leaguer be frustrated at striking out in the first game? No doubt she will, and some kids throw their bats and helmets and walk away miserable and dejected. Will your baby feel frustrated about putting herself to sleep? No doubt she will, and she will toss and turn and cry and throw a tantrum. Will our little leaguer finally acquire this new skill of hitting a ball? Absolutely. Will your baby learn how to sleep? Absolutely.

Should Parents Let Their Baby Cry? *Yes!*

The bottom line is that a baby will get frustrated and cry when learning this skill, but it won't be the last time that achieving a skill and frustration will go hand in hand. This crying is not due to pain or hunger or fear of the unknown, but is a way of dealing with the frustration of learning to fall asleep. Her crying may last for thirty minutes or for several hours. Whatever the length, the best advice is to allow the crying to continue; do not take the baby out of her crib. In fact, she will learn more quickly that she can fall asleep on her own without parental intervention if she is left on her own to figure it out. Crying will not hurt the baby physically or emotionally. Usually, babies will learn within a few days that their crying does not bring a parent and that they can fall asleep without parental intervention. Instead of seeing the crying in a negative way, I view it as a means to an accomplishment that only the baby can achieve for herself. While the baby is learning to fall asleep, both she and her parents are beneficiaries.

What Else Is Happening?

Sleep issues tend to be a major focus at four months, but babies at this age have other characteristics. Years ago, when babies were placed on their stomachs for sleep, they developed upper body muscle tone by pushing up and off the crib mattress. By four months, they could roll over, and every grandparent knows of this gross motor developmental milestone. Now that we advocate "back to sleep," with babies sleeping on their backs, babies are no longer rolling over at four months. Instead, since they are on their backs much more of the time, their arms and hands are freed up sooner. Today's baby may not roll over but she surely can reach out and touch someone. Hand-eye coordination progresses faster than it used to just because of a change in sleep position, and babies grab objects and bring those objects to their mouths with gusto.

At this age, babies are able to push off and bear some weight. They like to bounce on their legs in an adult's lap. In fact, this activity not only strengthens leg muscles, but also allows remodeling of those leg bones that were so curved in utero.

Also, placing babies on their abdomens for periods of time encourages development of the muscles of the upper body and shoulder girdle. This muscular development, in turn, promotes better head control.

What to Eat

Perhaps the most fun at a baby's four-month visit to the pediatrician is to talk about food and feeding babies. While various committees of the American Academy of Pediatrics differ on when to begin feeding, I think that four months is a very reasonable time to start. What evidence we have suggests that there may be fewer allergies and better nutritional benefits by beginning feedings at four months.

The exciting new information about feeding is that it does not matter what food you begin with and what order you need to follow. Feeding needs no rules, except the rule not to give honey until a baby is two years old. As said in an earlier chapter about feeding, the reason for this delay in offering honey has nothing to do with digestion or allergy but rather that honey may carry bacteria that make botulinum toxin. This toxin can be lethal to children under two years old.

Feeding foods to babies at this age requires a mushy-textured preparation whatever the food might be. Our ancestors most likely chewed on whatever they had to eat and then spit it out and fed it to the baby, similar to mother birds who feed their young in this manner. Abandoning all the former rules about which category of food or what color of food to introduce first and for how long means that parents can feed their babies whatever they are having for dinner. Puree some dinner food or, for convenience, choose jars of baby food. As long as the texture is soft, a baby can enjoy whatever food is offered.

Language Skills Haven't Changed Much

Since the earlier stage of cooing, the language skills of a baby don't seem to have changed very much. Some babies are becoming more guttural, but many just make their desires known with screeches and crying. Language is the highest cerebral function and obviously separates us from all the other mammals. One must be patient about the acquisition of language skills.

- Sleep can be an issue. Most babies have either acquired the sleep skill or are ready to be challenged. Allowing a baby to cry herself to sleep is not harmful and will bring more peace and harmony to any household.

- Encourage the gross motor skills of better head control and bearing weight. Some babies might roll over but not all do since we changed their sleep position.

- Those pesky infant rashes disappear, and baby's skin becomes baby soft.

- As for language, don't expect more than screeches, cooing, and crying.
- "Back to sleep" babies excel at the fine motor skills of reaching out and grabbing objects. Hand-eye coordination is ahead of schedule compared to babies raised on their stomachs.

Parent Lauren R. wrote,

Dr. Dan always took my calls and allayed my anxiety with humor. One particular time that stands out for me is a call I made to him when my son first learned to roll over. My baby was rolling himself in one direction in his crib and then would scream because he couldn't get back onto his original position. He would do this all night long and I was getting up, rolling him back, only to have to do that again and again. Having been rather spoiled by my son early since he had been a great sleeper, I wasn't used to getting up so often anymore.

I called Dr. Dan because I was distraught and exhausted, and I begged for THE solution. He listened patiently and then said, "You could always try duct tape."

I realized from this exchange that my son's behavior was yet another "phase" that he would outgrow and my best bet was to wait it out.

19

Fever, Infections, and Alternative Medicine

I went to college with every intention of becoming a lawyer. My dad was a lawyer and a judge in New York, and my older brother was also planning to become a lawyer. It was in our genes. By the time I was a junior in college, I decided to change my career goals. As I began my junior year, my older brother was selected for Law Revue at Columbia Law School. The entire family was thrilled by this, but for me, it presented a problem. I realized that I was not likely to achieve that degree of excellence in law. I had a learning disability that made reading difficult for me. If I had trouble reading English, I began to wonder how I would be at reading legalese. The answer in my mind was I would not be very good, and I should rethink my career goals. The decision process did not take very long. In my family at that time, the options were somewhat limited. You either became a doctor or a lawyer. If a lawyer I was not to be, then a doctor I must be. I went to my college adviser and told him of my change of plans. I needed advice on how an English major with an art history minor could go to medical school. I completed my degree at Columbia College with a whole lot of science classes crammed into the last two years. New York University Medical Center was willing to take a chance on an applicant like me, and I began a career as a doctor with a background in literature and art rather than science. That background has served me well as a clinician and a teacher.

Medicine Is Like Literature and Art

Fortunately for me, medicine turned out to be like literature and art. Medicine is based on our current scientific knowledge, but it is not practiced as pure science. There is a well-accepted distinction in the medical community that is referred to as the "bench" versus the "bedside." The "bench" doctors are the investigators who seek out the mechanisms of disease and try to determine the truth about biologic and physiologic processes. Science aims at the truth. It searches for the evidence that proves something conclusively. The bench is the laboratory work station where they do their work. They work very hard at all hours. Occasionally, they make a great discovery, but most of the time, they are searching for the truth.

The "bedside" doctors are those physicians and nurse-practitioners who try to take the knowledge from the bench and apply it to you as an individual. They see you in the office and take your calls in the middle of the night. They are there at the bedside when you are sick. They work very hard at all hours. Occasionally, they make a great diagnosis, but most of the time, they are also just searching.

In art and literature, there is no truth. There is rarely one interpretation of the meaning of a book or a renaissance painting. Medicine from my perspective is a lot like art and literature. There are many interpretations of the signs and symptoms. One must hear the entire story and take in the full picture before coming to some conclusion. The conclusion is rarely the only conclusion possible. This is the nature of art.

Second Opinions: Of Course

It is important as new parents that you understand the limitations of the provider in providing answers to your questions. Whatever the issue may be that we are dealing with at any moment, very intelligent people can come to very opposite opinions. When it comes to dealing with individuals, we are dealing with medicine as an art and not a science. We apply scientific information from the bench, but it is not always applicable at the bedside. Each baby is an individual, and much of our knowledge is based on statistics for large groups. Not every individual will act according to our statistics. What is good for the goose may not be good for the gander. In any given situation, the doctor and parent may not agree; and many times, the doctor and another doctor may not agree. This does not mean one side is right and another wrong. You need to have a working relationship not only with your doctor, but among yourselves as parents with everyone looking toward the best interest of the child. You and I as your doctor must also be willing to admit when the path we have chosen is not working for that child. This need not be an admission of stupidity but rather the wrong choice for that situation.

The Art and Science of Fever

Any temperature at or above 100.4 degrees Fahrenheit is considered a fever in the first year of life. This refers to a temperature taken rectally with a digital thermometer. Ear and forehead thermometers are considered to be inaccurate. They may falsely give elevated readings, and the consequence of that elevated reading may be an extensive workup for the infant that might not have been necessary. Fever is one of the four signs that there may be inflammation somewhere in the body (see later chapter about the immune system).

Fever is a flag being waved to let you know something may be amiss. Fever tells me, as your doctor, to put on my detective hat and try to identify the cause.

Fever under Twelve Weeks of Age: A No-brainer

For a pediatrician, fever in a child less than twelve weeks of age requires a certain response. Children in this age group are at risk for major infections for several reasons. First, their immune systems, though installed, are not yet fully functional. Second, they were exposed, during the birth process, to various bacteria that may have colonized them at delivery but do not become invasive until weeks later. Third, they are so young that, as a pediatrician, I cannot interpret whether they are acting normally. For instance, if they are sleepy, they could be ill or sick, but usually, they are simply tired. If they are irritable, they could be ill, but most normal babies less than twelve weeks old are irritable. Fourth, they have either received no immunizations or, at the most, only one shot, so they are at risk to a wide host of diseases. And finally, they don't have reserves to fight off infection. They need fluid and calories every three to four hours, and their metabolic rate is in high gear. Add to this an infection and their energy needs can be quickly overwhelmed.

Basically, it's just too difficult to tell how sick an infant in this age group might be or how quickly he can get in trouble in terms of his circulatory and metabolic status.

It, therefore, is a no-brainer to send these children directly to the emergency room. This age group will need more than just an examination to determine the cause of the fever. More often than not, this baby will need a blood count, a blood culture, a urinalysis, a urine culture, a spinal tap for spinal fluid examination and spinal fluid culture, and a chest x-ray. This is not fun for the baby or the parents, but it sure beats missing a major infection that, in this age group, might be life-threatening.

After this workup, the lab data is reviewed; and more often than not, we still do not know the cause of the fever. Although we are unsure at this point, the statistics clearly lean toward a virus as the causative agent. This is one time, however, when we do not play the odds because the risks are too great if we are wrong. Instead, we treat all these children with antibiotics while we wait for the cultures of the blood, urine, and spinal fluid to return. These cultures take up to three or four days, and during that period, we cover the remote possibility that there is a bacterial infection. This treatment is, at times, given in the hospital with intravenous medication, and at other times, the child is treated with intramuscular injections and allowed to go home. The choice is made totally dependent on the circumstances in each individual case. When a cause is discovered, then that definitive diagnosis will determine the type and extent of treatment necessary.

Fever: Over Three Months and up to Two and a Half Years: Not a No-brainer

There is a wide range of opinions on what to do for the child with a fever who is over three months and less than two and a half years old. First, what's special about this age group? Why do pediatricians focus on this age range? The answer relates primarily to the language skills of these children. They can't tell us what the matter is. They do not say, "Doc, my ear hurts" or "It hurts when I go pee." A major part of our assessment of how ill an individual may be relates to his mental status. Under two and a half years of age, that assessment is not always easy because we cannot hear what the child has to say. Older children make my assessment of fever easy. More often than not, they tell me what the problem is. Younger preverbal infants and children make pediatricians work harder for the answers.

However, the evaluation of these children is easier than those of children less than three months old. Unlike the child under three months of age, these children have a more mature immune system. They are not as metabolically stressed as their growth rates are slowing down, they are past the period of infections acquired at birth, and they have been around long enough so that one can have some sense of how normally or abnormally they are behaving.

History of a Moving Target

The evaluation of a fever in a child begins with the history and a complete physical examination from head to toe. Most serious infections will be detected at that point, or at least, the seriousness of the illness will be determined. The child's mental status may be confused, suggesting either severe dehydration, a metabolic abnormality, or an inflammation of the brain. His respiratory rate may be increased and his lungs not clear, suggesting pneumonia. He may have a rash or a barky cough that is typical of a given disease. He may have a pocket of red swollen and tender area of tissue that brings our focus to an abscess. In each of these instances, the further pursuit of the diagnosis and institution of treatment becomes clear.

However, he may have nothing, and there is the rub. What should one do with the perfectly normal child between three months and two and a half years who has a fever more than 102.6F and looks perfectly fine? Studies have been done in this group, and it was found out that if the total white blood cell count is more than fifteen thousand, then these children had a 5 percent chance of having a bacterium called Pneumococcus in their bloodstreams. Five perfectly normal-appearing febrile children out of one hundred were at risk for a serious disease even though they appeared normal. They had what we call an occult bacteremia. Bacteria were in the bloodstream and were being circulated around the whole body with the potential to settle in and damage the organ systems of the body.

The Immune System to the Rescue

All was not lost because, as noted in chapter 14, the immune system is ever vigilant. The studies showed that in four out of five cases of occult bacteremia, the immune system successfully destroyed the invading bacteria. Only one in one hundred children continued with bacteria in the bloodstream when untreated. However, that one child could succumb to meningitis or death. Therefore, pediatricians know that if the white blood count is elevated, they should obtain a blood culture to see if bacteria were present and, in the interim, begin antibiotics immediately to eradicate the possible risks.

Even though we know we are protecting only one child out of a hundred, no one should doubt that this is the proper course of action.

The Pneumococcal Vaccine to the Rescue: Maybe

With the introduction of the pneumococcal vaccine, opinions have begun to vary among physicians as to what to do with the febrile child who appears to be well. Some believe that for a vaccinated child, the risk of occult bacteremia is gone. Others believe that this is only true after the full series of four vaccines has been given. The series is not complete until fifteen months of age. Others believe that even though Pneumococcus may be gone, new strains of opportunistic bacteria may begin to cause the same disease.

In Boston, we are blessed with several major medical centers that care for children. Pediatricians at these different institutions have different protocols for treating febrile children who appear to be well; not all of these centers check the white blood cell count in such febrile children. They look at the same scientific evidence, but they do not see it the same way.

What's a Parent to Do? It's Better to Talk than to Walk

It is important that you choose a pediatrician whom you trust to help make the best decisions for your child. You need to be able to work together. If you disagree or are not sure, you and your physician have to make the effort to clarify what is going on. It is part of my everyday life to hear from a patient that her friend's doctor said one thing and I said another. Who is right? Many times we are both right because we have the evidence to back up what we said. Of course, the problem is which evidence we choose to believe.

You and I can disagree for the same reasons. We both choose what evidence we want to hear. What is important is a willingness to listen to the other side. If this discussion is not happening, then its time to walk and not talk.

Alternative Medicine: What Is the Evidence, and Who Do You Believe?

It amuses me that people like to talk about alternative medicine. Today, this is couched in terms of East versus West. I am asked during a prenatal visit, "What is your position?"

My position is very simple: there is no "ternative" medicine, for lack of a better term, that was not once "alternative" medicine.

What we do today for the treatment of many conditions is based on the observation that people with these problems seemed to do better in certain localities than in other localities. For example, people with "dropsy," heart failure today, used to seek alternative sources of relief by going to a town in France. After a while in this town, their fluid accumulation in their legs and shortness of breath improved. People thought it had something to do with the local waters. It had nothing to do with the water and everything to do with the local bakery. It turned out that the baker included in his bread a chopped up plant called foxglove. Years later, it was determined that a compound derived from this plant called digitalis was the cardiac stimulant that improved cardiac function and cleared the fluid retention in persons with heart failure.

Digitalis is now commercially manufactured and is definitely "ternative" medicine. Its roots, so to speak, were totally alternative. Obviously, any alternative medicine or approach, which over time proves to be effective, will be incorporated into what is established practice. I have no problem accepting, in regard to developmental and behavioral issues, that if what you first try as a corrective measure does not work, then do not hesitate to try the opposite. I feel the same way about many treatments. My own achy back has always responded better to physical therapy and chiropractic approaches than anything I was told to do by an orthopedist. On the other hand, the torn ligaments in my knee responded better to orthopedic surgery than anything I was told to do by my chiropractor or physical therapist.

So in answer to "what is your position," I believe you have to flow like water and bend like a willow. Even the "traditional" advice on hot versus cold for injuries, margarine versus butter for heart disease, fat versus carbohydrates for a better diet, lay in bed or stay mobile after a heart attack, isolate or mainstream the delayed child have done reversals during my career. We are back to my advice for my medical students. Question everything, and always wonder if the opposite of what we are thinking turns out to be true. This does not mean do not act and move forward. It means move forward with an open mind that, at a moment's notice, is ready to move backward.

Parent Judith R. wrote,

I remember Dr. Dan's patience in responding to my call at 3 am one morning, suggesting calmly that I put my toddler in a tepid bath (the water is neither hot nor cold but body temperature) and get in with her to allay her fears. Dr. Heller advised me that my daughter would much prefer being home with me and that the hospital staff would do a similar thing for a child with a fever of 104 degrees.

20

Six Months: Pursuing a Meaningful Relationship Already

The difference between playing and talking with a six-month-old baby compared to a younger infant is the newly acquired interactive component in the relationship. Younger babies clearly absorb visual, verbal, and tactile inputs and process that information. You need to talk, touch, and respond to your infant. However, as noted before, too much input may prove to be overwhelming for the immature nervous system. In the first few months, babies can easily become overwhelmed by too much stimulation. Their nervous systems are very immature, and infants are easily overwhelmed by too many inputs. Under six months, a baby may easily fall apart and cry uncontrollably when the sensory receptors cannot handle the inputs.

Babies **under six months** generally have an all or nothing approach to stimuli. They are fine, or they are miserable with few in-betweens. One response fits all situations. This single response limitation frustrates parents because parents sometimes find it difficult to understand what their babies are upset about. Babies have the same global crying response and total body fretfulness whether the stimuli is due to hunger, an itch on their buttocks, or a dislike of a color or odor. Of course, we assume that hunger or gas is the culprit, and when feeding and burping prove not to be comforting, we become aggravated. Nancy and I were no different than anyone else when we would ask our nonverbal infants under six months, "What do you want?" For all we knew, the answer might have been "A little classical music please. I'm tired of listening to the Beatles."

One Exception to the Rule

One day, when Marissa was four months old, I was holding and watching her in her room. She was at that stage where she had discovered her right hand and was staring at its beauty and subtle movements about eight inches from her face and just off to the right. At that moment, Nancy returned from a prolonged shopping trip and came into the house. The front door slammed shut, and the noise caused Marissa to have a startle reflex. Her right hand moved out and away from her visual field and came back in a reflex manner next to her body. As she settled down, her head moved, and her eyes stared into the space where her hand had been. Her lips curled down into a frown, and she began to cry. She could not find her beautiful hand. It had somehow disappeared, and she missed it immediately. Nancy came upstairs and responded to her cry with the comment, "Lucky I came home. You sure sound like you're hungry."

This was one of the few times that I knew better: She was not hungry. She was crying because she lost her right hand.

If only I really knew what was behind most crying, I would be a very smart parent and pediatrician. More often than not, we do not have a clue why our babies were crying. We just have to take a good guess, and if at first we don't succeed, try and try again.

Won't You Come Over and Play?

Six-month-olds, on the other hand, are beginning to develop both interactive skills and modulated responses to different stimuli. Everybody loves a six-month-old, and six-month-olds love everybody. Six-month-olds are prepared for and enjoy all types of input. By six months, babies are better equipped to integrate multiple inputs and, more importantly, respond to those inputs in a modulated fashion. Instead of "one cry fits all situations," giant steps are occurring relative to socialization and personal interactions and measured responses. This is a very exciting time for everyone. The baby is beginning to show some personality. Smiles at this age are definitely not due to "gas." Laughs are for real, and everyone senses it. Playing peek-a-boo or bouncing the baby is fun both for the baby and the grownups. Six-month-old babies can respond to grandparents, aunts, uncles, friends, and siblings. Figuring out "What do you want?" is becoming less frustrating.

Babies also are interested in everything at this age. You do not need to buy any special toys. The inside of a roll of toilet paper is as intriguing as an expensive gizmo. Sight, sound, and tactile inputs are being absorbed and integrated as the infant's brain continues to develop.

Motor development is also moving ahead now at leaps and bounds. A six-month-old can reach out and grab objects and transfer them, at times, from one hand to the other. Some babies are able to maintain a sitting position briefly at this age. Rolling over becomes a commonplace event.

Taking Control

A six-month-old can accept or reject food, grab and observe a toy, shake or silence a rattle. In other words, she has options other than just crying and being fretful.

Babies are learning to control themselves and, to a limited degree, their environment. It is important to respond to these interactive behaviors and enjoy them. It is equally important not to become ensnared on the STEPS issues, which begin to take on real meaning at this age. STEPS refers to the control issues involved with sleeping, talking, eating, peeing, and stooling. For a six-month-old and her parents, the STEPS issues that become real are related to sleeping and eating. Not only is the baby beginning to be interactive, but she is discovering that she controls what and how much she will eat and when and how much she will sleep.

Speaking of Control: You Cannot Lose What You Never Had

As a parent, you cannot make your baby eat or sleep, and you should avoid getting into a conflict on these issues. During a scheduled mealtime, don't try to force your baby to eat. However, don't be forced to feed her outside of regular mealtimes either. You will serve approximately 19,710 meals between now and your baby's eighteenth birthday. Missing a few of those will not matter. I have yet to see a baby starve herself by skipping meals or missing between-meal snacks.

A Brief Aside about Eating in the Long Run

In fact, obesity has become the number one eating disorder among older children and adolescents. Are the seeds of this problem sewn at this early age? We do not know the answer. What we do know is that the advice we have given over the past forty years may have resulted in the increase of anorexia, bulimia, and obesity. My opinion is that we give far too much advice about feeding. Parents should be less anxious and concerned about what and how much is fed and be more on encouraging when it comes to fitness and physical activity.

For American children, eating has almost become the major daily exercise. We would be well advised to spend as much time improving our fitness as we spend sitting and eating. When you add up three meals a day and the snacks between meals and treats before bedtime, we take about six time-outs each day to eat. Unfortunately, the only muscle group to benefit from this type of exercise is the maseter muscles of the face.

Our focus on feeding and eating has a second negative consequence for the child and the parent, and that is feeding often proves to be an exercise in frustration. Like it or not, your baby decides what she wants to eat as well as how much and how often she partakes. This choice does not always quite mesh with parents' notions of what is good or not good. I urge you to realize sooner than later that you do not control the eating habits of the child, nor should you let the child control you. The focus of feeding is to sustain life. The focus of life should not be eating. Let your baby choose her foods and stop when she seems satisfied. Try not to make eating a full-time, all-day event.

The Bumper Sticker: If Your Not on Your Feet, There's No Reason to Eat

Even at this age, going outdoors and using one's body are critical to mental and physical development. As adults, many of us are forced into sedentary jobs; and while our income may increase, so does our girth. Our physical fitness does not benefit. I am upset when parents tell me that the "baby hates being on her stomach." The parental response is to immediately pick up and hold the baby, thereby denying their child the chance to develop upper body motor strength. It is almost as if we are promoting lack of fitness and strength. Remember that with exercise, we build our muscles, we strengthen our bones, and we burn off fat. That is a perfect recipe for health whether you are six months old or sixty years old.

Slipping on the Sleeping Step

As with eating, sleeping is another area that highlights the lack of control a parent might feel. Don't try to force your baby to sleep, but don't be forced to stay up or get up when she does not want to sleep. Certainly by six months, your baby's brain is well developed enough to have normal sleep patterns. The number one reason for a "poor sleeper" is lack of behavioral training and not physiologic or medical reasons. As noted earlier, your baby, not you, needs to learn how to fall asleep (see chapter 18). As with many other acquired skills, the baby may have frustrating moments during the learning process. She will learn to read and write and hit a baseball with your help. However, in the end, she will have to step up to the book or the pen and paper or the plate and accomplish the task by herself. You control the bedtime, and she controls the sleep time. Most babies are well established in their ability to sleep by six months. For those who are not sleeping, six months is the time for them to step up to the plate and accomplish the task. Usually, one or two nights of crying will solve the problem, and everyone will be happier for this achievement in the long run. The baby will be pleased she can control her sleeping, and the parents will be happy to sleep.

Nancy's Voice: Please, please, please go to sleep.

Our first child was a marvelous sleeper as a young infant. She began to sleep for seven hours at night when she was only five weeks old, and by the time she was twelve weeks, she was sleeping for twelve hours. I thought that this pattern would continue for a long time. For weeks, I had nursed her to sleep, carefully putting her in bed so as not to wake her, and tiptoed out of the room. I even feared that the creaking of her door as I closed it would awaken her. That never happened, but when she was five months old, she resisted our routine. When I put her in her crib, her eyes would fly open, and she would howl in protest. Allowing her to cry seemed much too hard on her emotions and mine, so I brought her downstairs to be with us whether we were having dinner, watching television, reading, or studying. On some of these evenings, she would play happily or be content in her infant swing; but on too many occasions, she would be fussy and irritable. No amount of comforting helped.

Dan was still a resident in pediatrics and had no idea what to do. I sought advice from a friend with older children. She encouraged me to let my baby cry herself to sleep. My friend warned me that I might have to let Marissa cry for even as much as two hours. I resisted the advice for a couple more weeks, but finally, out of desperation, I gathered my courage. I picked a night when Dan was on call at the hospital because I figured that together, our resolve might crumble. On that night, I nursed Marissa as usual, put her in her crib, and said good night. Of course, she immediately began crying.

I hurried to my bedroom, closed the door, and turned up the volume of the TV until I could not hear Marissa's cries. I do admit that I turned down the volume and opened the door every ten minutes or so (or maybe every few minutes). My heart was breaking, but somehow, I steeled myself to close my door and turn up the volume again. Finally, finally, finally, after what seemed like an eternity but was actually only sixty minutes, Marissa stopped crying and fell asleep.

The next night, I was better prepared since I knew that she could fall asleep on her own. She was better prepared too because she only cried for thirty minutes. She had obviously learned a lesson from the evening before. On the third night, she cried for only fifteen minutes, and on the fourth and subsequent nights, she did not cry at all. I felt great; in later years, as I reflected on that experience, I realized that I had learned the most valu-

able, and perhaps the most difficult, parenting lesson: setting limits on behavior, even when children are very young, is critical to the well-being of both parent and child.

I'm Hungry: Now What Shall I Eat

Thirty years ago, babies began to eat mashed and soupy solid foods at six weeks of age. As they grew older week by week and month by month, they learned to eat more textured foods. By the time these babies reached six months of age, parents could throw caution to the winds and feed them table foods.

In fact, the six-month visit back then was fun for the parents because they could stop buying prepared baby foods in the form of custards and mashed meat and vegetable or could stop spending time to puree home-cooked foods; instead, they could begin serving their baby whatever was being served to the rest of the family. I have a collection of pictures from those days showing babies eating their first unadulterated, homemade table foods. These six-month-old babies are eating barbequed spare ribs, cucumber, french fries, scrambled eggs, mixed vegetables, and corn on the cob; I have one picture showing a baby from Iceland gnawing on a smoked sheep's head!

Parents of my patients are awestruck when they see these pictures. They first wonder how these babies can accomplish this feat and then quickly realize that our foremothers and fathers did not have various-staged, prepared baby foods or food processors to make their own. Our ancestors, from the beginning of time, chew on food and spit it out to feed their babies. My patients' parents who come from less well-developed parts of the world tell me that even today, the mother's mouth, rather than a Cuisinart, is the site of most baby food preparations. Admittedly, some six-month-old infants still prefer everything mashed and enjoy being spoon-fed, but others are quite capable of picking up pieces of food and gumming the food down all by themselves.

Over the past two decades, the advice has been to delay all solid feeding until six months of age. The same rules about infant feeding were carried forward from six weeks to six months, and babies began feeding on mashed or mushy foods. In this country, no one was prepared to give barbequed ribs as the first meal. Today's advice allows us to introduce foods at an earlier age once again and return to those wonderful days of yesteryear where six-month-olds could feed themselves (see chapter on the history of feeding).

Giving Your Baby Control over Eating: Multiple Benefits

Allowing a baby to feed herself has two distinct advantages over the spoon-feeding of all foods. First, the baby will choose what she likes based on her tastes and her texture preferences. Your baby does not have to eat everything or like everything. Infants grow quite successfully on diets that are unique to certain parts of the earth. Just because we have every type and variety of food does not mean that your baby has to eat them all. Variety may be the spice of life, but everyone does not like spices.

Second, a baby will decide when she is satisfied and sated. Most infants, if left to their own choice, will not overeat. Most parents, on the other hand, will usually overfeed. We often tell our kids, "Take just one more bite" or "You must finish everything on your plate," as if this extra amount had any nutritional value. Keep the long-term perspective in mind. The extra bite just gets stored as fat, and enough extra bites foster obesity. As noted above, the single greatest eating disorder that confronts pediatricians today is obesity. Some evidence suggests that fat cells multiply in children under the age of two in response to the demands of the body to store fat. These fat cells remain with an individual for her entire lifetime. The child who carries fewer fat storage cells with her on the journey of life may be at an advantage relative to weight control issues and longevity later on.

There is nothing inherently wrong with fat, carbohydrates, and protein. In fact, they are the stuff we are made of. Your brain and central nervous system need fat (and this is even more true for babies). You use carbohydrates to fuel your energy requirements, and you need protein to build muscle and body tissues. Babies are growing rapidly and need these three nutrients. This is not the time for a restrictive low-fat, low-carbohydrate, or low-protein diet. This is the time not to overfeed for the sake of feeding. It's a fine line to know what and how much to feed. Generally, I like to trust the baby to make these decisions more than the parent. Success is judged at the scheduled well-baby visits. The height percentile of the infant determines the appropriate weight. The generally accepted rule is that an infant should have a weight that is either one standard deviation above or below their height percentile. I think the baby who is at the lower weight percentile is going to be better off in the long run. I also think that the rate of growth is more important than the actual percentile. Weight that is either increasing or decreasing faster than the normal percentile curve needs evaluation. On the other hand, a weight that is low but following a normal curve is not a cause for alarm.

You Have the Right to Remain Silent: And Indeed She Will

At six months, a baby has come a long way with her fine and gross motor skills and her personal-social and interactive abilities. Language acquisition, on the other hand, takes a longer period of time. In fact, at six months, our baby needs only to have progressed from cooing sounds to more guttural noises. Guttural sounds are formed in the back of the mouth by adjusting the vocal cords, which are in the upper airway. At six months, we begin to hear sounds like *gaga*, *jahjah*, and maybe, just maybe, *dada*.

Of course, fathers all go wild over this *dada*, but rest assured, it is a sound with no meaning. Many mothers ask why we do not hear any mama sounds at six months. The answer relates again to brain immaturity. To say *mama* or *baba*, we have to close our mouth so that our lips are pursed together.

Dada is an open mouth sound and requires only a one step of vocalization. These early vocalizations represent the building blocks on which a real language can be constructed. Sounds like *mama*, *papa*, and *baba*, on the other hand, require a two-step vocalization process. You need to first close your mouth and then make the sound. These closed-mouth sounds are major clues that your baby's cerebral language skills are developing normally and at a higher level of differentiation. Closed-mouth sounds will develop between the sixth and ninth months of age. It will still be quite a while before language, as we know it, begins to reveal itself, but it is very important to respond to these vocalizations and "talk" with your infant.

- Gross motor milestones—Sit and roll over; Wow, your baby is finally catching up to my German shorthaired pointer. He did this at one week of age.

- Personal-social milestones—She has a sense of humor and plays interactive games. This is someone with whom you want to have a long-term relationship.

- Learning to modulate responses and easier to identify needs.

- Language—Working on the project, but we still have a long way to go.

- Fine motor—Look mom, I can feed myself.

- Taking control of sleeping and eating—not you but rather the baby.

21

Asthma, Allergy, and Eczema: The Magical Mystery Tour

My brother Bob would sneeze a lot and have itchy eyes. My mom took him to the allergist who did eighteen skin tests over his back and arms. The tests showed he was allergic to dust mites, molds, ragweed, grasses, dogs, cats, and about eight other things. A "special" desensitizing antiserum was then ordered for Bob, and he had to get a weekly shot throughout the rest of his childhood and continuing on until college.

When I was about thirteen, I made the great mistake of sneezing once too often. Mom called the allergist. He told her it was not necessary to skin test me because most likely I would show the same sensitivities as Bob. Therefore, it was good enough to give me the same desensitizing antiserum that Bob was given. Just like Bob, I became the victim of a weekly injection that was to continue throughout my childhood.

Of course, both Bob and I continued to sneeze; but at least, my mom felt she was doing something. When I finally went off to college, my mother made arrangements for the antiserum to be mailed monthly to the school and kept properly refrigerated. Out of either rebellion or good sense, I never went over to student health to get my all-important antiallergy shots. After two years, somehow my mother was informed that there was a refrigerator filled with my unused allergy shots. She was pretty annoyed that she had paid for all this mystery material but forgave me when I told her I had stopped sneezing anyway.

Of course, the allergist would argue that Bob's desensitizing antiserum was responsible for my recovery. I would argue that my recovery was directly related to me not using Bob's desensitizing antiserum. This all occurred over forty-five years ago. The sad thing is that we are no better off today in our understanding of these seasonal allergies than we were back then. Importantly, allergies and asthma account for an enormous chunk of our health-care dollars, and one has to question whether the expense of diagnosis and treatment are worth it. Despite all the headlines, I do not think we have progressed very far in our evidence-based approach to allergies and asthma. Before you and your child become embroiled in the issues of milk allergy, food allergy, seasonal allergies, environmental allergies, and the whole area of asthma, lets take a look at what we do know.

Cow's Milk Allergies and Soy-based Formulas: Timing Is Everything

When it comes to allergies, you are guilty until proven innocent. It amazes me how many bottle-fed babies are discovered to be allergic to cow milk-based formula on the second or third day of life. The diagnosis is usually based on the fact that the baby spit up his one- or two-ounce feeding. Doctors and parents are quick to blame the formula and change to soy. The fact that a normal full-term baby requires no intake on the first three days does not affect the decision making. The fact that the baby still has mucus and amniotic fluid in its gastrointestinal system for the first few days is not considered. The fact that whatever you might put in on the first two days might be regurgitated does not matter. The fact that the immune system takes seven to ten days to mount an antibody response is ignored. No, in many people's minds, the cow's milk must be guilty of causing the vomiting, and it must be a manifestation of milk allergy. No one wants to admit that any volume of any liquid might be vomited up immediately in the first few days. This is not an allergy. This is a pediatrick.

Baby Jennie is a case in point. I was off for a vacation last fall and returned to meet baby Jennie, who was two weeks old when I returned. Baby Jennie's parents decided to bottle-feed her, and she began on a perfectly fine cow's milk-based formula. She vomited this formula twice and was declared by the covering doctor to be allergic to milk. The standard knee-jerk treatment of this condition is to go on soy-based formula, and so baby Jennie was changed to a soy-based formula before she was twenty-four hours old. She vomited again on her second day of life, and the covering doctor was contacted. He changed her to a fancier predigested formula. She was on her third formula before she was forty-eight hours old. On her hospital discharge, it was noted that she had spotty rashes on her chest and back and mild perirectal excoriation, both of which are perfectly normal.

However, this prompted the doctor to change her formula one more time to another that is basically made up of amino acids and predigested fats and carbohydrates. When I meet Jennie, she was two weeks old and on her fourth formula. She is already above her birth weight, which is unusual. In fact, she is totally normal, and you would think everyone would be happy. Unfortunately, the parents are not happy. The specialized formula she was on was not only hard for the family to obtain but was extremely expensive. These are not the richest people on earth, and their insurance company is not, surprisingly, balking at paying for this formula.

I found nothing in Jennie's history to suggest any problem with any of the formulas. Normal newborns spit up, and that was all Jennie had done. We stopped the fancy formula and returned to the first cow's milk formula, and needless to say, Jennie thrived.

She did fine because there was nothing wrong in the first place. Given several days to clear mucus and digested amniotic fluids, any formula will be retained better. It was not the formula switches that benefited Jennie, it was a tincture of time. Jennie's story is not unique. It is estimated that about 30 percent of babies get switched to soy formulas for supposed milk allergy or sensitivity, and yet almost all these babies have no problem with milk products when they are older.

Where Did All the Allergies Go Long Time Passing?

Where did all these milk allergies go? How did these children stop being allergic? True allergies are mediated by the immune system. The immune system has a memory that lasts for a lifetime. Did the immune system in these supposed milk allergic children develop some type of immunologic Alzheimer's disease?

I posed this question to several top allergists at different Boston hospitals that care for children. One thing is perfectly clear. There is a wide range of opinions on this topic and very little real evidence to support any one opinion. Generally speaking, when the evidence is clear-cut, everyone agrees; so it is not surprising that in the area of milk and food allergies, where solid evidence is lacking, many opinions flourish. One specialist summarized this "allergy" situation in an easily understood way. He said, "The generation of specific allergic responses to foods in most cases is an aberration. Most of us do not develop pathologic immune sensitivity to foods. Our immune system knows not only how to distinguish self from non-self, but also dangerous from non-dangerous. So it is appropriate to make an antibody response to a virus or a bacteria but inappropriate to make one to egg or milk."

It is more likely and logical that there was no milk allergy to begin with. I would bet if we began all bottle-fed babies on soy formula that by day three we would be switching them to cow's milk-based formula and declaring they were all soy allergic. In essence, we misuse the word *allergy* when a baby vomits its formula or gets a rash on its face or buttocks. Babies vomit and get rashes with or without drinking milk or eating certain foods.

The cow-milk-to-soy-milk substitution that supposedly is a remedy for milk allergy in newborns is also a favorite trick for the treatment of colic that arises after two weeks. Fussy babies are frequently changed from cow's milk to soy between two and eight weeks of age for the treatment of colic. Here again, it is the timing and not the formula that makes the difference. Colic is a predictable behavior with a predictable time course. Any change in routine that I suggest during this period, I can credit as leading to the disappearance of the colicky behavior. It is not the formula change but time that improves the situation. Colic is not due to a milk sensitivity or allergy to milk. Again, if I started all babies on soy formulas, I would bet that by three weeks of age, 30 percent would be switched to cow's mild-based formula with the argument that their irritability, poor sleep, and colic were due to a soy allergy. When there is no science, opinion and conjecture reign, often not to the benefit of the baby.

Solid Feedings and Food Allergies: OJ Found "Not Guilty" along with Co-conspirators Chocolate, Nuts, and Strawberries

You would not believe the number of foods that parents tell me their child is allergic to.

I have some children who, it would seem, could not survive on this planet if indeed what the parents call allergies were actually real. As with the issue of formulas, we misuse the term *allergy*. In actuality, only 3 to 5 percent of children have food allergies characterized by anaphylactic shock, gastrointestinal hemorrhage, or severe hives. Many four- to six-month-old children are called allergic because they get a rash on their faces or have diarrhea or are irritable in association with solid feedings. Unfortunately, many four- to six-month-olds get rashes, have diarrhea, and are irritable all by themselves. In fact, if you wiped your breakfast, lunch, and dinner on your face and drooled on your body, you might get rashes on your face and body as well. We would not call this an allergic reaction but rather the consequence of being a sloppy eater.

The picture is further complicated by two additional factors. First, many viruses can cause both nonspecific rashes as well as hive-like allergic rashes and yet be hardly noticed as a symptomatic disease. Second, the immune system takes seven to fourteen days to respond to foreign materials. The rash you see today may have been a consequence of an illness or food that was encountered up to two weeks earlier. This obviously makes it harder to pinpoint the possible culprit and be definitive as to the cause. It's all too easy to start blaming many innocent bystanders for the rash on your baby. In actuality, most of these rashes are nonspecific, meaning, we do not have a clue as to their real cause but can be confident that they are of little consequence.

True Food Allergies Are Not Too Subtle

If you have ever seen someone who had an anaphylactic reaction to a bee sting or food, you would never forget it for the rest of your life. Perfectly-normal-looking people will suddenly have a concerned look that distances them from whatever they are doing. They may complain of a "funny" feeling in their lips or upper throat. Their breathing becomes more rapid and then more difficult. They become air-hungry and fight desperately to move air into their lungs. If you are the observer, you will call 911 and wonder what else you can do to help.

Anaphylaxis is not hard to miss. A less dangerous but far more common allergic reaction to foods and other allergens is the development of urticaria. Urticaria is more commonly know as hives or allergic rash. It is recognized by a central wheal or raised area with a flare of redness in a circular pattern. These circles may be as small as a quarter of an inch or very large. Urticaria usually occurs all over the body and can be very itchy and uncomfortable.

As noted earlier, almost any allergen may trigger urticaria, including viruses, medications, foods, inhaled particulate matter, and topical exposures. With so many causes, it is not at all surprising that I rarely can figure out the cause of this systemic skin rash. The insulting agent could be something that was encountered two weeks ago or a reexposure to it on the day the rash appears. On top of the difficulty of timing, the insulting agent need not continue to be present for the rash to continue breaking out. There are cells in your skin called mast cells. These cells release histamine when certain antibody-antigen complexes stimulate them. Histamine causes the rash we call hives, and at the same time, it stimulates other mast cells to release more histamine. This reaction can go on literally for days or weeks even though the initial causative agent is long gone from your system.

Unfortunately, since we eat three meals a day and snack so much, food always seems to have a temporal relationship to the development of the rash.

Stopping the reaction is fairly easy. Antihistamines stop the release of histamine and end the rash, or steroids can be given to stabilize the mast cells and prevent further histamine release. Determining the cause of the reaction is not so easy.

State-of-the-Art Allergy Workups: Not So Stately

My allergy specialist colleagues all agree that a history of breathing trouble or ana-phylaxis is evidence enough of an allergy. Beyond that, they seem to be of two different schools on how to evaluate the possibility of a real allergy. One school believes in skin testing, and the other in blood testing (RAST tests) for specific allergens. Both methods have significant false positive results. Positive skin tests are seen in children with no allergic symptoms, and the same is true of positive blood tests. Many argue that skin tests cannot be accurately interpreted in children under three years old and, some say, under seven years old. This fact does not seem to deter allergists from performing these tests and pursuing these work-ups. Despite the fact that there can be as high as a 30 percent disconnect between positive skin tests and actual symptoms, judgments about your child's allergic status are based on these tests. The state of the art is not so stately.

Ultimately, the best test is a challenge test done in the doctor's office where immediate treatment is available should a major reaction occur. A food challenge is just what it sounds like. The suspected food is given to the individual and then is observed for any reaction. When adults are questioned about food allergies, about 20 percent believe they have an allergy to one or more foods. However, only 1.4 percent of these individuals show positive findings on a food challenge test. Generally, it is hardly worth doing a food challenge in a child who has had a major anaphylactic reaction. A food challenge in this instance would be danger-ous. That child is allergic whether skin or blood tests prove it or not.

Outgrowing Allergies: Patience Is a Virtue

Why do so many infants and children outgrow their food allergies? The most likely answer is that they never had allergies to begin with. Alternatively, some children are not really allergic to the foods but rather to preservatives, colorings, and flavorings that are chemical additives to the foods. A third possibility is that the immune system matures in its control mechanisms over time. The good news is that very few children actually have food allergies despite being labeled as such in infancy. It really does not matter what foods you introduce and in what order (see chapter on feeding infants).

How to Reduce the Risk of Food Allergies: The Early Bird Gets the Worm

When I began to practice thirty years ago, the theory was put forward that food allergies were due to the early introduction of solid feedings. Over the years, solid food feedings were delayed from six weeks to twelve weeks and ultimately to six months. The concept was that a more mature bowel would be better equipped to block foreign proteins from passing through the bowel wall intact. There were also certain foods that were considered highly allergenic such as eggs, strawberries, chocolates, and nuts. These foods were not introduced until much later.

What's Food Got to Do With It?

Maybe the food has nothing to do with these reactions. For example, a recent article in the *New England Journal of Medicine* presented some evidence that the oils in lotions used to treat eczema might be absorbed through the skin and cross-sensitize the infant to peanut oils. The suggestion was that the allergy to the peanuts had nothing to do with eating the peanuts but everything to do with the exposure of the skin to oils similar to peanut oil used in treating the eczema.

Today, more and more evidence is accumulating that earlier exposure to allergens may decrease rather than increase the likelihood of allergies. Children raised on farms have seven times less likelihood of asthma than children raised in the city. Children in homes with pets are twice less likely to develop allergies to animal dander than those in homes with no furry pets. Houses that are dirtier and have dust mites and other small organisms give rise to less asthmatic children. What is going on here that might explain these paradoxes?

You Won't Believe It, but Here Is the Crappy Answer

One current explanation is that the immune system of the infant and young baby makes different antibodies depending on a number of environmental factors. The immune system is capable of making different classes of antibodies. There are allergic T-helper cell antibody responses and nonallergic T-helper cell antibody responses. The antibodies made in response to a foreign material may be the type that stimulates histamine release and an allergic reaction, or they might just attack the foreign protein and not trigger an allergic reaction.

More and more evidence is coming out that the type of antibody response may have something to do with the excrement of animals large and small. In the stool of all animals are bacteria that release a toxin called endotoxin. Children in homes that are dirtier with dust mites or on farms with animals are exposed to more endotoxin and are definitely less allergic in to dust.

If this proves to be true, then the great rise we have seen over the years of allergies and asthma may be the result of our avoidance of early confrontations. Stated differently, we ought to introduce foods and expose our children earlier to supposed allergens. My own experience over the years is that the delay in exposure has certainly not reduced the number of children with asthma and allergies. The rates of asthma are definitely on the rise. We also know that the foods we claimed were allergenic here like peanuts and chocolates are not allergenic in other countries where they are introduced earlier. It would appear instead of helping to reduce asthma and allergies, by avoidance we have only contributed to the problem. As Marie Antoinette one said, "Let them eat cake."

One Food Rule Remains: Don't Get an Egg on Your Face

Eggs remain as a potential food allergen risk, and the current thinking is to delay eggs in specific instances. If both parents or one parent and one sibling have known egg allergies, then the advice is to delay introducing eggs to your baby. Some say to delay eggs for a year, and some for two years. A side issue related to eggs is whether or not infants suspected of egg allergies should receive the MMR vaccine (measles, mumps, and rubella) or influenza vaccinations. Both of these vaccines have components requiring growth on chick embryos. Oddly, the answer is different for each vaccine. The MMR has presented no problem even for egg allergic infants. The influenza vaccine, on the other hand, should not be given to an infant with egg allergy.

Asthma Issues in the First Year of Life

Keeping pace with the rise of allergies in infants and children is the concomitant rise of asthma. Asthma goes by many names, including wheezing, reactive airway disease, tight chest, bronchiolitis, and restrictive lung disease. They all mean that the airways are narrowed down and restrict the easy flow of air in and out of the lungs. Just as roses by any other name smell the same, so too asthma by any other name is just as scary. And scary it is. If you want to experience what it feels like to have asthma, just try and breathe through a straw or open a ball point pen and breathe through the channel that holds the refill. Within a minute, you will be struggling to move enough air through that narrow channel. The soft tissues in you neck and between your ribs will be pulled in with each inhalation because you cannot move air in fast enough to fill the vacuum. We call these unusual chest movements retractions. You will begin to breathe faster to make up for the restricted movement of air. As time goes on, you will tire out; and if you don't get rid of the straw or pen, you will not survive.

Asthma Is Not Pretend

A child with asthma is doing exactly that, but he is unable to remedy the narrowing because it is happening within his lungs. He will need medication to dilate the airways and allow air to move in again, and he will need medication to stop whatever triggered the process in the first place. If his asthma is severe, a call to 911 is necessary in order to find competent medical personnel that can help to return the respiratory system to normal. Along with seizures and croup, asthma is one of the things a baby or infant might have that scares both parents and pediatricians. Trouble breathing is not an issue that can wait until morning. The causes of asthma are many, but the treatments are relatively few and generally effective. Most of the causes trigger a sequence of events in the airways that lead to respiratory distress. For many years, it was argued within the medical community that children under one year could not have "true" asthma because they did not have smooth muscles in there airways that had to constrict to cause the restriction. Today, we know that children can have reactive smooth muscles in their airways and manifest all of the signs and symptoms of adult asthma. Viruses such as respiratory syncytial virus (RSV or bronchiolitis) are the most common cause of asthmatic symptoms in infants and young children. Many children have this illness in the first year of life and never wheeze again. However, some children seem to have bronchiolitis more than once. It is now clear that some of these children are not having recurrent episodes of a viral infection but rather have sensitive airways that react to various irritants or stimuli by constricting. Causative factors can be environmental such as smoke or other air-borne toxins in homes, foods, molds, viruses, heat, cold, and humidity. In fact the possible triggers are too numerous to mention. Everyone agrees that there is more asthma now than twenty-five years ago. The real question is why asthma is on the rise.

Extra, Extra: Asthma on the Rise Because of _____ (You Fill in the Blank)

Every week, in the journals I read, I find articles talking about asthma and its causes. Everyone seems to have an opinion on this issue ranging from pollutants to additives in our foods to preservatives and household cleaning products. Last year, I went to a grand round at Massachusetts General Hospital given by Dr. F. Martinez, an allergist and asthma specialist from Arizona. He presented his research about kids growing up on farms versus kids from the city and the relationship of their exposures to animals and dirt to the development of asthma. His research clearly demonstrated that there are less incidents of asthma among children with more exposures to endotoxin early in life than among those who did not. He found, as noted earlier, that exposure to endotoxin from animal feces affected the immune response. Those exposed to endotoxin were more likely to make non-allergenic antibody responses than those who were not exposed. Since endotoxin is a by-product of bacteria in the stools of animals, it begins to make sense that growing up around animals may be protective against having allergic responses.

As I have noted before, when I am not sure what to think about a medical topic, I try to think what my caveman ancestor did in a similar situation. How did our early caveman deal with asthma? Likely, if he had asthma, he died! He did not have the rescue bronchodilator drugs available or the controller drugs to block a recurrent episode of wheezing. He could not call 911. That our species has survived suggests that there could not have been so much asthma ten thousand years ago. What is different between that world ten thousand years ago and our world today? Clearly, our caveman grew up among animals and, secondarily, around endotoxin. They very likely had less asthma because they were exposed to the poop of animals and their living quarters were not clean.

Pollution Must Be the Answer

We hear daily that the air is not good, and pollutants are spewing forth from our industrial development. There is truth in this statement, but pollutants are not new. Dinosaurs once populated this planet, and the current theory is that a meteor struck the earth with such force it filled the atmosphere with dust so thick it blocked the sun and choked all living things to death. Now that is what I would call pollution. Earth is a great mixing bowl. It rotates around its axis every single day, and wind and water currents mix the planets resources on a continuous basis. Trees in one part of the planet give off oxygen to fill in the gaps created by highways and parking lots. And just as the good oxygen gets distributed all over the planet, so do the evil pollutants. Yet the rates of asthma are not the same all over the planet Earth. Rates are higher in the industrialized nations even during the time when we are moving our industries abroad. Rates of asthma have been increasing over the last decades despite increased, though inadequate, measures to control pollution.

I am not convinced that pollution is the answer.

Our Lifestyle Must Be the Answer

When I heard Dr. Fernandez talk, something began to click relative to my caveman ancestors. Children growing up on farms and in rural areas and our caveman had something in common. They both spent time outdoors. They both interacted early with their environment out of necessity. Today's city dweller has a much different lifestyle.

We live in homes and apartments with our windows sealed shut to save on our heat in the winter and our air-conditioning in the summer. We drive our cars with the windows closed for the same reasons. In fact, we spend relatively little time in touch with our natural environment. Is the result of this lifestyle that we do well when we are in our own little controlled environments but fall apart with asthma and allergies when we step outside into the real world?

Like everyone else's theory on this subject, mine may be no better or worse. Unfortunately, we have no real evidence to support or substantiate a claim for why asthma is increasing. No one can dispute that we are spending more time indoors, and what little science and experience we have would suggest that outdoors may be better.

Eczema: the Third Conundrum of Infancy

While it is easy for me to say your child has eczema, it is not easy for me to say why. Along with allergy and asthma, the origins of eczema are not clear, leaving the topic open for many advice givers and sellers of remedies. Eczema refers to patchy areas of dry, scaling, itchy patches of skin on the flexor surfaces of the arms and legs and around the face. While many say it is due to food allergies, especially to milk and egg products, it almost always appears before any solid foods are ingested.

Some say it has a very strong genetic component. I can vouch for the fact that Asian babies, for example, have much worse eczema than Western infants. Apparently, this is true whether they are raised in Asia or in the United States. That is not to say that environment doesn't influence the severity of eczema. And indeed, environment, once again, may be the main factor.

More of the Same Crappy Answer

A recent study published in *Pediatrics* looked at the exposure to endotoxin and the development of eczema. Sure enough, just like with the asthma story, exposure to high levels of endotoxin seemed to be protective against the development of eczema in the first year of life.

Many things that take place in the first year occur in proximity to other events. We give an immunization, and the baby has a rash a week later; and we wonder if the two events are connected. We start food, and the baby has a rash; and we wonder if the two are connected. For years we have associated asthma, eczema, and allergies to the types and timing of the introduction of food. We observed that asthma and eczema occurred in the same timeframe as the beginning of feeding. We delayed feedings until six months in order to decrease these problems and were disappointed to find these problems increasing. We wondered why children in Asia who had an entirely different introductory diet did not have as much asthma and allergies. Could it be the food had nothing to do with these problems?

Tricked Again

The endotoxin story, though incomplete, is putting a brand-new light on these associations. The advice about delaying foods, avoiding pets, and keeping our windows closed to have a clean house had nothing to do with the rate of asthma and eczema. In fact, we very likely made the problem worse. This is not a unique story in medicine. For years, we said that ulcers in adults were due to a type A personality and stress. Antacids and surgery were common treatments. When research showed that a bacterium, *H. Pylori*, was the cause and antibiotics were the cure, many of us were skeptical. Time has shown that, indeed, our skepticism was unwarranted.

Remember, the Ugly Duckling Turned into a Swan

The one nice thing I can tell to parents whose child has eczema in infancy is that they will outgrow it over time. Each year, the eczema usually gets better such that by five years of age, it stops being a problem. This improvement very likely relates to a maturing of the immune system. Fortunately, for these children, they are able to suppress the allergenic immune response over time.

On the other hand, some eczema may have a different etiology. Jessica is a patient of mine whose eczema was very bad throughout her infancy and childhood. I always felt sorry for her and the discomfort she suffered not only from the physical appearance but also from the pain of chronic itching. Neither I nor specialists in dermatology and allergy really could offer much more than symptomatic relief. Then, when she was thirteen, she began having her menstrual periods; and to my amazement, her skin cleared up. Clearly, the changes in hormones associated with adolescence did more than all our earlier treatments. Eczema remains a mystery to me. We are slowly learning about some of the pathways that lead to this skin disorder, but it appears that no one answer fits all the cases.

Food allergies are rare, rashes are not.

- Children outgrow their food allergies either because they never had them or their immune system matures.

- Endotoxin used to be part of environment. Not all toxins are bad.

- When it comes to food, there are no rules except for eggs and honey. That's all folks!

- Earlier feeding is advice worth heeding.

- Visit the earth early. It's on the other side of the window. See it, breathe it, and touch it; and you may have less asthma and allergies.

- Eczema is not forever.

22

What's in a Name?

We gave considerable thought about what to name each of our three children. At nine months of age, we were surprised to realize that we had given them another name (and the same for all three). We began calling each of them "Oh no" in turn. "Oh no" rapidly becomes the form of address that most parents use when talking to their nine-month-to-one-year-old child. "Oh no" is said so frequently that I am convinced that most babies begin to think this is actually their name.

You will hear yourself say, usually in a raised or anxious tone of voice, "'Oh no,' don't touch that socket," "'Oh no,' that oven door is hot," or "'Oh no,' look at the mess you have made." From a child's viewpoint, the phrase "Oh no" rapidly becomes either meaningless or, at minimum, unclear.

What's a Child to Do?

As part of the learning process, a child utilizes as many of her senses as possible to understand what is being taught. For example, babies learn by mimicking what they see and hear. They see and hear you say please and thank you or observe the goodbye kiss to a friend or loved one. They also see the response of the other person involved in this interaction.

However, when it comes to the concept of no, a baby finds herself handicapped. When did you last have dinner with your spouse and say to him, "Oh no, look at the mess you've made"? Very likely, the answer is not lately. The point is that the baby has no examples to mimic when it comes to this "oh no" statement. Lacking a model on which to program a response, infants are left to their own devices as to how to react. Some children smile or laugh and proceed with the actions they were engaged in. Others give a soulful look and begin to cry. Still, others become angry and upset.

The situation is further complicated for babies because we use the "oh no" expression for both behavioral corrections as well as for warnings of physical danger or harm.

What's a Parent to Do?

You need to distinguish for the infant the difference between "Oh no, that's dangerous" and "Oh no, that's not acceptable" behavior. Of the two, the concept of what is dangerous must be addressed first for the safety of your nine-month-old. And the way to do this is to make clear what is dangerous.

Dealing with Danger

Parents must make a clear verbal distinction between the dangerous oh no's and the social oh no's. Dangers or threats to your child necessitate a direct and active approach. If a baby reaches out to an electric socket or an open oven door or any other possibly traumatizing item, her parent ought to yell, "NO, DANGEROUS!" and then rush over and pick the child up. The baby may be so scared by the no-dangerous yell that she cries, but that is perfectly fine. You want to stop her in her tracks if she is approaching danger, and you want her to know you are coming to her aid. If, on the other hand, you calmly say "oh no, that's dangerous" in a pleasant tone, I will guarantee you she will not think this is very unusual and may reach out and touch the socket or hot oven door. The receptive language skills of a nine-month-old are well ahead of her expressive skills. She will understand by tone and facial expressions the differences you are conveying about what is and is not dangerous. Basically, you must distinguish for the nine-month-old what is truly physically dangerous from what is just an annoyance that is not physically harmful.

Dealing with Behavioral No-noes

You have many options when coping with social and behavior no-noes. Avoiding conflicts is probably the best way to reduce the number of times one says no in the course of a day. In other words, if you don't want your child to play with your Ming vase, move it out of reach. Expect that she will not be the neatest eater at this age and that playing with food can be great fun. Limit the no-noes around food issues to those that really bother you. And, most importantly, be willing to provide an example for her to mimic.

Remember that a firstborn child has only her parents to use as an example for her responses. A second or third child has the advantage of observing not only parental behavior, but also the behavior of her older sibling. Especially with a first child, set an example by making a few social and behavioral mistakes yourself. Your baby can derive two benefits from this type of action. First, she can observe your response when you do something wrong. Second, she won't feel that she is the only one in the family being criticized all the time. For example, Nancy or I would purposefully knock over our almost empty coffee cup during a meal. We would then come out with the inevitable "Oh no, look at the mess you made" comment. The klutzy perpetrator of this faux pas would quickly grab a napkin and proceed to clean up the mess and say, "I'm sorry." All this occurred in clear view of our child. Over time, she began to reach for the napkins when the issue was what to do about a mess. As parents, recognize areas where your child has no siblings or peers to help guide her response.

During my internship training, a favorite expression of physician supervisors was "see one, do one, teach one." This phrase related to the performance of procedures on patients. I did not intuitively know how to perform a spinal tap. A supervising resident explained to me the various steps of a spinal tap as he performed the procedure. The next time we had a patient who needed a spinal tap, I would actually perform it. At that point, in theory, I could teach a younger doctor in training.

In actuality, most interns see several repetitions of a given procedure before doing one; gaining the confidence to teach the procedure is acquired with time. The principle though is quite applicable to teaching a child and watching her attain a skill. As in the case of the medical intern, if your child does not observe a particular response to a situation, she may have a harder time figuring out which response is the most appropriate.

NINE MONTHS: Mobility, Agility, and Liability

Beginning at nine months, babies add a new ability to their ever-growing repertoire of tricks: mobility. Babies begin to figure out how to get from one place to another, and the methods are variable. Some roll over and over while others drag themselves. Usually, babies develop some type of efficient crawling. Some babies are clever enough to persuade their parents to buy them walkers so they can skip these primitive forms of locomotion. One way or another, babies will begin to explore their environment, and they will explore it with gusto.

The Earth Is Flat, and You Can Fall Off the Edge

Frequently, I receive an emergency call from a parent whose child just fell out of bed or rolled down a flight of stairs either on her own or in a walker. With their newly acquired mobility, babies reach the edge of their world and actually fall off. Fortunately, most children seem to survive this adventure unscathed. Nature must have known that falls would be common as children learned to coordinate their gross and fine motor movements. Due to the flexibility of the joints and bones, much of the trauma is absorbed and dissipated. Heads actually are particularly well designed to protect the most important organ, the brain. As stated in an earlier chapter, the bones of the skull are not solidly fused together during infancy. During the birth process, the non-fusion of the cranial bones allows the boney plates of the skull to ride over one another so a baby's head can be delivered. These bones remain in a non-fused state for almost three years of age. The non-fused bones of the skull act as a safety mechanism against potential injuries from trauma.

Built-in Safety Devices

If we hit our heads, the soft tissues of our brains may be shaken up and swell. This swelling occurs within our skulls, which are like sealed containers. Pressure develops on the brain tissue, and we will exhibit symptoms of brain swelling. We become confused, dizzy, and nauseated. We may begin to vomit and become unconscious. A baby's brain, on the other hand, may swell; but instead of meeting the resistance of a sealed skull, the bones will move outward and release any pressure that is generated. In this regard, babies and toddlers actually cope better with head trauma than older children and adults. Babies do not usually become lethargic, dizzy, and nauseated because the bony system of their skulls allows for the dissipation of pressure. This system is not foolproof, however, and if your baby incurs significant head trauma, your pediatric healthcare provider must evaluate her injury. If your infant is unconscious, do not hesitate to call 911 for emergency services. However, if your baby cries immediately, she most likely would have escaped serious injury, but you should consult with your pediatric office or health-care facility.

Reducing the Risks of World Discovery: Sounds Simple

The point is that with mobility come liabilities. Babies who are mobile cannot be left unattended by parents or caregivers for even one second. Nor is it ever safe, at any age, to leave a baby on a bed. I have seen many supposedly non-mobile babies learn to roll over in a bed and end up head first on the floor. Some parents object to putting their babies on the floor, but even if the floor is cold or dirty, it is a far safer place to leave a baby, who cannot fall off a floor. Obviously, safety is important, and planning ahead is the best preventive measure to avoid a problem.

Maybe It Is Not So Simple

The issue of baby proofing is similar to many areas in pediatrics; everyone has an opinion, and the choices are left to you. Just as every coin has two sides, every issue in child rearing seems to have at least two differing proponents. For example, should you have baby gates in your home? The answer would seem to be a resounding YES, and yet views vary widely. Some well-respected pediatric development specialists recommend baby gates at all stairways to avoid potential falls; one must provide a safe environment. On the other hand, other equally well-known pediatric development specialists recommend against baby gates on the theory that those gates restrict a child's natural desire to explore the universe; those specialists argue that you should be observing your child at every minute and that gates only provide a false sense of security. Should you have socket safety plugs? The standard advice is to install socket plugs throughout your home so that your mobile nine-month-old will not go sticking his finger or something else into one and be injured. And yet there are no socket plugs at grandma's house or in the supermarket or in an airport waiting area. Do socket plugs at home lead parents to be less vigilant of this danger in other places? Similar arguments arise over locking up kitchen cabinets and moving the furniture.

"Whither thou goest, I shall go"

My own experience has led me to believe that the best protection against most dangers is being constantly vigilant. Like it or not, you must keep track of your roaming infant. You either follow her where she goes, or she must accompany you wherever you go. If you need to use a bathroom, then your baby should come with you. You cannot leave her in a "safe" place. Mobility has its risks and benefits, and you have to try to make the best choice possible when it comes to a "safe" environment.

"The best-laid plans of mice and men often go astray"

I remember the day we brought Marissa home from the hospital. The welcoming committee included our dog and two cats, and we were ready to begin our new lives as parents. As we sat in the living room while Marissa nursed, Nancy saw our beautiful slate cocktail table in front of the sofa. That table had been one of our possessions for over seven years and never drew much attention. It had served the very useful function of holding newspapers and snacks during parties and as a place for me to rest my feet. That was before Nancy's transformation into a new mother. In the eyes of maternal Nancy, the table was a danger. She envisioned Marissa walking and tripping and smacking her head on its edge. She told me it had to go immediately. Marissa was less than a week old as I carried this very heavy slate coffee table down to the basement. That table was banished for the potential harm it might cause our daughter.

Two and a half years later, we were in the kitchen. Nancy was reading a book to Marissa at the dinner table, and I was washing dishes. The dishwasher door was open.

Marissa climbed down from her mother's lap and toddled into the kitchen. Why she tripped, I will never know, but she did trip as she had tripped without incident numerous times before. Unlike those times, however, she tripped into the dishwasher and cut her lip. After we returned from the hospital where a surgeon stitched our daughter's lip, I went down to the basement, retrieved the heavy slate coffee table, and reinstalled it in our living room. It wasn't Mr. Table in the living room with the fall; rather, it was Mrs. Dishwasher in the kitchen with the trip.

Accidents Happen

Clearly, one cannot anticipate every possible accident, or no more accidents would happen. My seven-year-old daughter, Sara, wearing brand-new patent leather shoes, slipped on a hardwood stage floor as she approached a piano during her recital. She caught the edge of the piano stool with her eyebrow and began bleeding all over her favorite party dress. Who would have thought you could get a hockey injury at a piano recital?

Many Choices but Few Good Answers

As a parent, you are caught between a rock and a hard place when deciding what is best for your child. The stories above relate to physical accidents and traumas. However, mental and developmental issues also should be considered. The early exploration of the environment by a nine-month-old is only the beginning of a life of moving out and discovering new things in new places. Each exposure of your infant or child to new sights, sounds, places, and things is a learning experience. An infant's brain needs these exposures to fully develop, a process that does not end in infancy. As a parent, your challenge is to provide a secure environment without limiting that environment so much that your baby's growth, both physical and mental, is inhibited. You have made choices during all of your life. However, making choices for a child becomes a much greater burden. Your choices will affect not only you but also another person. This is part of the fun and the challenge of parenting.

Let's randomly pick the issue of daycare to illustrate the difficulties of parenting. Should a child begin a daycare experience at this age? From a safety perspective, one child with one parent observing her is probably safer than a child in a daycare with one teacher observing four children. From a learning and developmental perspective, a child at home with one parent is less stimulating than being with one adult and three other children. Of course, no perfect answer exists; but with a nine-month-old, questions abound.

Psychological Parental Paralysis: More Common Than You Think

The best advice is not to become paralyzed and overanalyze every issue. All too often, I see parents struggling over issues; they ask me for "the right answer." But all too often, there is no right answer.

For example, I am frequently asked if the baby who wakes during the night should be brought in bed with the parents or made to stay in his crib. There are arguments on both sides. Historically, everyone always slept together. I was impressed, when I visited Plimouth Plantation, to see a small room with a large fireplace and, placed directly across from that fireplace, a large rope-strung hay-covered bed with sheet on top. The guide explained that in 1620, the entire family slept together for reasons of warmth. The parents, children, and indentured servants all huddled together. The concept of a separate nursery for children comes much later and is reserved for those who can afford to heat multiple areas in the home. So what is the correct answer to the question? Partly, it depends on the infant involved. Some babies are wonderful to snuggle up with and sleep peacefully through the night. Our own Sara slept with us as a young child and continued to sneak into bed with us up to age six. When she stopped, I asked her why, and she said she was too tired to come join us. Other infants can, quite frankly, be annoying when you try to sleep with them. They may toss and turn and pull you or your pillow, and this makes for an unpleasant night's sleep for everyone. And co-sleeping with very young infants poses a real danger of suffocation.

In the end, do not become psychologically, parentally paralyzed. Make a decision, and give it a try. You will find that it may or may not work and make adjustments accordingly. Remember that these decisions are affected not only by you and your spouse, but in her own way, your baby has a "say" in the matter.

Any experience your child has will enhance his knowledge base. Feel comfortable to try an approach; observe how your baby responds. As with many issues in pediatrics, there is no one correct answer to the questions above. Some babies thrive in one situation, and some in another. Fortunately, as time goes on, it becomes easier to read the signals from your baby as to his likes and dislikes. Both of you will make adjustments over time, and both of you will learn over time.

The Thrill of Having a Nine-month-old: A Two-way Relationship

The gross and fine motor skills of a nine-month-old move forward rapidly. Expressive language development may not be obvious. Receptive language skills are not only apparent but are also contributing to a significant interchange of ideas between parent and baby. Nine-month-olds are becoming more adept at understanding what their parents are saying. This understanding goes beyond the tone and facial expression and into the actual meaning of the words being spoken. Your baby is now really observing how you as parents relate to each other. They notice your pleases and thank-yous and will mimic them later in life. They are observant of visitors and storekeepers and other children. They are literally on the fast track over the next several months in understanding and using all of this verbal and social information.

But don't expect a specific *mama* or *dada* for a while. Expressive language comes after the receptive language. Take advantage of the acceptance of receptive language. You don't have to speak baby talk at this stage. Speak as you would to any person, and if the family speaks more than one language, use them all.

Nine months is also the time to begin reading to your child and enjoying a good book together. Nine months is the right time to allow her to observe interchanges and interactions of persons; such observations assist babies in developing social skills and in dealing with similar situations later in her life. She is rapidly learning not only how humans interact with language but also how they socially interact.

Preemptive Advice on Eating and Sleeping

Almost all parents report, at the nine-month visit, that they are having trouble with feedings. Their babies are eating less and becoming fussy and picky. Yes, babies are eating less but not because they are fussy or picky. The fact is all that babies' growth slows dramatically as they approach one year of age. Babies eat less because they are growing less. Do not worry about this decrease in food consumption because it is normal.

Coinciding with their decreased growth, babies are teething at nine months. Teething may add to fussy periods and decreased interest in solid foods, but again, this is perfectly normal. During this period, many babies begin to wake up every night, and parents are quick to blame teething for this change. I do not think teething is related to most nighttime awakenings. Teething may affect the ability to fall asleep but usually not the ability to stay asleep. During periods of teething, the gums ache. In the daytime, a baby's interactions with her environment distract her from her focus on her gums. However, at bedtime, as the lights are turned off and distractions disappear, her brain will focus on the discomfort in her gums. Once she falls asleep, her cognition of this discomfort is diminished, and she should not be waking up due to teething. If her gums are so inflamed that she does wake at night, she usually has a fever, and the episode only lasts for one day or so.

Then why do babies wake in the middle of the night, night after night, at this age? To be honest, I do not know. I am unwilling to cast the blame, beyond one or two nights, on their teeth; certainly, they do not have ear infections or other illnesses unless they have fever. The most reasonable explanation is that the waking up is another patterned behavior. A baby quickly learns that if she awakens and cries in the middle of the night, people come to care for her. She may be held and rocked or given an extra nursing or bottle as a reward for awaking. If you have a baby who awakens on a nightly basis, your first course of action is to check for a fever or other problems. If you do not find a problem, then you should go in and give a quick pat on the back and leave. She will probably cry, but you need to set limits for her by not responding to her entreaties. While that may seem harsh, parents who have tried this approach report to me that after a few nights, their baby resumes her normal full night sleep pattern.

Nine-month-old Babies: Learning at the Speed of Life

- Your baby is thinking and processing information and using all her sensory receptors in a much more organized manner. Take advantage and input, input, input.

- Your baby understands more than you might think and is learning the skills to have social interactions.

- Your baby will slow down on food consumption as her growth rate slows down.

- You need to accept the difficult but rewarding job of parenting—making choices for your child's development. In many instances, no "right answer" exists.

23

Dr. Dan's Advice on Favorite Topics

Dr. Heller's original thinking and unconventional wisdom was, of course, not limited to the first year of life. He was intent on sharing his insights and advice on every aspect of a child's growth to adulthood—from potty training to drug use. Here are some notes he made outlining those topics and, fortunately, the recollections of families who took his advice to heart.

His first outlines for his thoughts included pithy one-liners on a variety of topics that he called the catch-22s of pediatrics.

The Missing Catches Before and After Catch-22

I was in high school when my cousin, Joseph Heller, authored his book *Catch-22*. *Catch-22* referred to the craziness of flying a bomber in a war zone. You could not fly if you were crazy. Of course, you had to be crazy to fly a combat mission. If you realized that you were crazy to fly, then in fact you were not crazy; and therefore, you could fly. Although I was only in high school, the idea of "catches" resonated with me.

In pediatrics, we have many catches. Here are the first twenty-one.

- Catch #1: You do not actually have a specific due date. There is a thirty-day range.

- Catch #2: You are pushed to make milk on day one, but you can't until day four.

- Catch #3: You are told your baby needs milk on day one. He doesn't because he has plenty of fluid.

- Catch #4: Jaundice in the first few days has nothing to do with the mother's lack of milk. It has everything to do with the maturity of the baby's liver.

- Catch #5: Low blood sugar in the first few days has nothing to do with the mother's lack of milk. It has everything to do with the baby's endocrine system.

- Catch #6: Colicky behavior is normal behavior and needs no treatment.

- Catch #7: Gastroesophogeal reflux is normal and needs no treatment.

- Catch #8: Staying indoors and not socializing is bad for the mother and the baby.

- Catch #9: It is a trick to make you think you control the baby's sleep.

- Catch #10: It is a trick to make you think you control the baby's talking or crying.

- Catch #11: It is a trick to make you think you control the baby's eating.

- Catch #12: It is a trick to make you think you control the baby's peeing.

- Catch #13: It is a trick to make you think you control the baby's stooling.

- Catch #14: Delaying solid food until six months may not be good for the baby.

- Catch #15: Never put a baby to sleep in his bed when he is asleep.

- Catch #16: Never give solid food to a baby when he is hungry.

- Catch #17: If a baby is becoming fat, begin feeding him solid foods.

- Catch #18: If you want to avoid allergies, face the allergens early on not later.

- Catch #19: Walk away, not toward, discipline problems.

- Catch #20: Since languages are harder to learn later, why not learn a few now.

- Catch #21: There is no need to have a book on pediatrics.

- Catch #22: Reserved by Joseph Heller.

And here are twelve more catches for good measure.

- Catch #23: Don't buy a humidifier. Open a window to humidify a room.

- Catch #24: Don't hire a lactation consultant before there is a lactation problem.

- Catch #25: Don't use a breast pump in the hospital. Give your baby a chance.

- Catch #26: Don't rush to buy soy formula. It may have a downside.

- Catch #27: Don't believe in ear infections with no fever.

- Catch #28: Don't forget to have life insurance.

- Catch #29: Don't forget to have a life!

- Catch #30: Don't delay or avoid immunizations.

- Catch #31: Don't desire to be on antibiotics.

- Catch #32: Don't avoid controller medications for asthma.

- Catch #33: Don't worry so much about the rare diseases and neglect the common ones.

- Catch #34: Don't think it is cool not to use a car seat or have a kid in the death seat.

The Slippery Steps of Parenting

In his notes, Dr. Dan wrote,

The slippery steps are five areas in which parents and children come into major conflict. Why? Because, in each and every area, whether you are dealing with an infant, a child, or an adolescent, you cannot win because these areas are not within your control as a parent. Whole books are written about these issues, and the fact is you can save your money. You don't control your child's **S**leeping, **T**alking, **E**ating, **P**eeing, or **S**tooling; and the sooner you figure that out, the sooner peace will come to your house.

The Slippery STEPS of Talking

Eighteen-month-olds may be struggling over control issues, but their language skills are above and beyond what you might think. Most eighteen-month-old children actually understand almost everything you say. Receptive language skills are remarkable at this age even if there is an exposure to more than one language. Some eighteen-month-olds may be more expressively verbal than others at this age. They may blurt out ten words or more and attempt to mimic sounds and parts of words even if the pronunciation is not correct. Others may be the strong, silent type. They comprehend what you say, but they do not verbalize. They point at objects and want you to tell them what it is, but they may not repeat the words until they are comfortable they will get it correctly.

Spitters and Sitters: Not Everyone Has Something to Say

I categorize children in terms of their verbal language patterns into the "spitters" and the "sitters." The typical "spitter" repeats words immediately but not necessarily correctly. They point to the refrigerator and you say *refrigerator*. They then spit out the word *ator*. You realize what it means, and they add it to their vocabulary. The typical "sitter," on the other hand, points to the refrigerator; and you say *refrigerator*. They then sit and say nothing. They may point at the refrigerator over a period of weeks and hear you say the word over and over again. Finally, when they are comfortable they have it right, they will say *refrigerator* in a clear and correct manner. As to why in regard to language some kids are comfortable to "spit" and others to "sit," I have no idea. I have been the proud parent of both types, and I firmly believe it is the child who decides when he will talk, how he will verbalize, and in what way he will say words. You cannot force expressive language or control it, and any attempt on your part will be met with frustration.

What you need to do is be active in talking and reading to your baby. You need to follow those pointing fingers and try to identify the object that is the focus of your child's attention. Say the words that you think he is trying to acquire, and do not get concerned if the response is that of a "spitter" and not quite correct or that of a "sitter" and nonexistent. As a pediatrician, I do not expect a two-word phrase until your child is two years old. I do expect to see receptive language skills improving all the time. When you ask an eighteen-month-to-two-year-old, "where is daddy" or "where is your bottle," I fully expect a look in the right direction or a movement to the object. As with many skills, the language skills will vary with numerous other factors. A baby's expressive verbal skills will be affected by the baby's birth order, home care or daycare, mono- or multilingual family, and other factors. As noted elsewhere, language sets us above all the other mammals; and its acquisition and successful use takes time.

The Slippery Step of Eating—Issues: One Year and Onward

Almost every mother of a one-year-old and onward complains to me that her child is a "poor eater." The desire to have a "good eater" seems to surpass any other accomplishment. Indeed, the issue of eating surpasses the issue of toilet training; and both, unfortunately, surpass the issue of talking and fine motor development in most people's minds. Why did we become so fixated on this eating thing and is it normal to be a "poor eater"?

The answer to the second half of the question is "Yes, it is normal."

In fact, infants begin life with a period of rapid growth that starts at full speed and drops off by two years of age to a slow and steady growth rate. A child will gain about three pounds of weight per year from age three to ten and yet will easily gain three pounds of weight in the first three months of life. Our babies gain from twelve to fourteen pounds in a year and then drop to a dismal three pounds per year. No wonder that moms think their children have become "poor eaters."

As to the first half of the question—why did we become fixated on eating?—the answer is not so clear. Two generations of Americans have seen world wars and other conflicts, and the take-home message relative to eating was that big fat babies seemed to survive famines and food deprivation better than skinny kids. If you emigrated here from Europe or Asia during a war time, you knew this to be the case. A good fat, pudgy baby became a sign of good parenting and good providing. Just like a private home and a two-car garage, a fat baby was a sign of success. Economic success was reflected in our possessions and our fat babies.

Unfortunately, from a health perspective, fat babies may not reflect success. Our bodies are somewhat driven by the demands placed on them. We are born with a certain number of fat cells to sustain a source for calories. Over the first two to three years of life, our bodies are able to make more fat cells if the need for more fat storage is created. The total number of fat cells in turn seems to drive our appetites. In other words, the more fat cells we have, the more fat cells we have to feed. The "poor eater," who is able to grow at an appropriate rate, ends up better off in the long run by having fewer fat cells to feed than the "good eater." It is more important to be a "good grower" than a "good eater."

Your well-child visits are scheduled in part to ensure proper immunization but equally important to ensure proper growth. Growth is not determined by daily checks on intake but by weight gain over time. Your visits are scheduled according to this fact. At first, visits are every two to four weeks because growth is so rapid. The visits then fall off to every three months, then every six months and, finally, yearly because growth slows. Just as with certain investments, there is nothing to gain by checking the stock value on a daily basis; rather it has to be done over time. Growth is a parameter to be checked over periods of time and not to be concerned with from day to day.

Another common question is "what should I feed my child?" or "shouldn't he get certain vegetables and a 'balanced meal'?" Probably more has been written on these subjects than the print is worth. When I was first trained in pediatrics, we used one set of rules; and now I am advised to teach a different set of rules. The bottom line is that there should be very few rules.

Clearly, different people in different countries and with different cultures feed their children differently. In 1988, the *New England Journal of Medicine* published an article called "Paleolithic Nutrition" by a physician and anthropologist, Bruce Konner. No other food advice has had as much influence on me as that article.

In summary, Dr. Konner pointed out that our caveman ancestors were hunter-gatherers and ate what they could find as they followed the herds of reindeer across the earth. They had no time to raise crops in one spot or eat farmed vegetables. Instead, they ate the roots and berries they found along the migratory trails of the meat sources that they followed. Of note is that the natural meat sources they ate were 3.9 percent fat since they were not farm raised. Today, our farm-raised meats are almost 40 percent fat in comparison. Our ancestors ate natural fish, which, unlike farm-raised ones, are also low in fat. Milk and milk by-products were not a part of the diet. Probably any self-respecting caveman seen grabbing an animal's teats and drinking its milk would have been viewed as a bit strange. Water was the natural liquid to drink as it is today for every mammal on the planet, except for us humans.

The truth is that there is no special diet for humans. We are well provided for by the earth with three food types: carbohydrates, fat, and protein. Arguments can be made for which is the best of each of these categories, and we can debate whether some are really better than others. However, the bottom line is there are just these three; and in the end, we need all of them. Without fats, our brains do not grow and develop. Without carbohydrates, we lack quick energy sources; and without the essential amino acids found in proteins, our bodies cannot build and replace our tissues.

Many pediatricians, nutritionists, and dieticians give very specific instructions about diets. They lay out exactly how much and the type of vegetables, meats, fish, and carbohydrates that your child should consume. When I first trained, I accepted this advice. Then the advice changed. Butter prevailed over margarine, and 40 percent fat in the diet dropped to 30 percent. One has to wonder why we keep changing our advice.

More importantly, I realized that it was the child who made the ultimate decision as to what to eat and not the doctor or the mother. My partner for many years gave mothers specific instructions on the "how much" and "what to eat" side of things. I watched as many mothers fought their children over eating according to these supposed scientific rules; I realized as I watched that the losers of the battle were going to be the mother, doctor, and nutritionist. Bobby Sands (an IRA member who went sixty-six days without eating to pressure the British government), Ghandi (who changed the course of India by eating or not eating), and Sakarov and Dick Gregory (who affected Russian and American foreign policies respectively) have all shown that food can be a weapon. Giving a child of one year a weapon as powerful as eating or not eating is not in the best interest of the parents or the child.

As noted earlier, people of different cultures eat different things. Obviously, there cannot be one diet that fits all children since that one diet does not exist in all parts of the globe. It was impossible for our own ancestors at Plymouth Rock to have green vegetables during that first winter in 1620. It is equally impossible for us today in New England to eat green vegetables in the winter, except for the fact that we can import them from South America. Are they really necessary? No. Are they good or bad? No. We get back to our need for fat, protein, and carbohydrate. Give us this day our daily bread, a source of carbohydrate. This is a land of milk and honey, our fat and protein and more carbohydrate. No mention is ever made of green vegetables.

Let's get back to the basics. Years ago, researchers studied the food behaviors of ten-month-old babies. The babies were presented with a tray divided into thirty-six sections. That tray included vegetables, sweets, meats, fish, etc. The babies in the study were given the same tray for each meal over a two-week period. The study showed that at no given meal did a baby eat the official percentages of fat, carbohydrate, and protein. In fact, over no given day did the babies balance their diet according to "rules." However, over a period of ten days, those babies did approach a balance of the three food types.

The best advice I can offer you is to trust your child. Most children, if not pressured, forced, cajoled, or tricked, will grow quite well without any battles. Most children will balance their intake because that balance is driven by internal physiologic mechanisms rather than preconceived notions and psychiatric biases about food.

Ghandi won, Dick Gregory won, Sakarov won, and your child will win a food fight. A good parent will provide food. A child will choose what he/she wants. I know children who ate only pasta from age one to twenty-one with occasional trials of other foods. They have grown well. I have patients who, because of kidney or gastrointestinal disease, need to be on restricted diets; and they have grown well. Food advice is not worth all the time and effort we put into it.

This food issue is really a huge one. I am convinced that when we diagnose a twelve-year-old with anorexia or bulimia or obesity, we are discovering the "fruits" of our obsession about food. The net result of all our food and feeding advice over the last fifty years has been a nation obsessed with food. Bookstores are loaded with books about food (how to prepare, how to serve, how to eat, which are best, the best diet, the least fat, the least carbohydrate, the all-protein). Before recent years, those who preceded us didn't have the luxury of so much advice and so many books. How did our species survive for many thousands of years without all this advice? Very simply, the answer has to be that the advice is not needed. Eating is basic, and feeding our babies and children does not require a book or advice. Trust your child and forget about the "rules."

The Slippery Step of Pooping, Potty Training and Constipation

Parent Ned W. wrote,

> We were worried about our toddler's irregular bowel movements and thought maybe she was constipated. With usual parental anxiety, we asked Dr. Heller. He explained that originally Moses was passed down 11 not 10 commandments. The 11th commandment was, "Thou shall poop everyday."

Dr. Heller told us that since obviously this was a commandment widely dismissed by people, Moses eliminated it from the list, and we would be wise to do so as well.

As a psychotherapist and supposed child development specialist, I was taken by the wisdom of this advice—and the genius of its delivery.

Parent Courtney H. wrote,

At our one year consultation, Dr. Heller said, "Last time I checked on college entrance exams, you will be asked, 'Can you read well? Do you speak a foreign language?'—The colleges certainly do not ask if you are potty trained—DON'T WORRY about when that happens—I <u>promise</u>—it will."

Parents Judith and Robert R. wrote,

At one well visit, when we were expressing our frustration in toilet training our son, Dr. Heller was, as usual, wise and funny. My son, at age 3.5, was adamantly refusing to use a toilet, demanding we offer him a diaper when "the need" arose. Dr. Heller smiled and said, "Don't worry. He won't go to Harvard in diapers."

Parent Carolyn L. wrote,

I miss Dr. Heller so much; there is a huge hole in all of our lives.

I am thrilled that you are going to publish his book, and would stand in line for hours for a copy of my own. I want to share the sage potty training advice I received in 2002 from Dr. Heller.

Our first discussion regarding our daughter, Lindsey, was early in 2002. This was our preliminary discussion, things to think about when potty training. To frame the discussion of when to start the training, he asked me a question: "On average, how old do you think children are when they are potty trained?

I replied, "Three."

Dr. Heller retorted, "Three what?"

"Three years," I replied.

"Well, you are close with the number, but the age is actually 3 months."

"Three months?!? How can that be?" (I'm wondering where I went wrong. For that matter, where all my friends who are mothers went wrong! How did I not know this. My curiosity was piqued.)

Dr. Heller explained, "Mothers in India, China, and Africa take their tiny infants down to the river and stroke the inside of their babies' legs to prompt the babies to go potty at rivers edge. We in the United States live in a modern society with modern conveniences like disposable diapers, pull up training pants, and running water in our homes. The average potty training age in developed countries is much higher than in developing countries. And part of the reason OUR mothers potty trained us so much earlier is because they were washing all those dirty diapers at home."

Imagine that! Now Dr. Heller had me thinking globally, but acting locally.

Next he turned around to rummage through one of his file drawers in his desk and was mumbling to himself, "Now where are they?...... Oh Yes! Here they are!"

He put three forms on his desk in front of me and said, "I have here the applications for Harvard, Yale, and Duke University, three very fine institutions of higher learning. You will notice that there is no question or check box on any of these asking if the applicant is potty trained."

We shared a smile and a chuckle. More importantly, the overall concept and urgency of potty training really came into focus for me. Dr. Heller had just given me an interactive, informative, and hilarious education. And, in an age of goal-oriented parenting, he delivered a very important message: they ALL get there in their own time. He went on to give more specific instructions, most of which I have since forgotten because these the main message was so artfully delivered.

Six months later, after Lindsey had been potty trained for a few months, she regressed to holding on to her potty when she took the big leap and began pre school. Distraught, I called Dr. Heller's office. (Another AMAZING thing about Dr. Heller is that he would sometimes take calls during the day! So I waited on hold, and after a few minutes he picked up the phone. Instant answers and gratification.)

I told him about the situation, and he immediately yet calmly said, "Just put her back in diapers."

"But, Dr. Heller, I KNOW she knows how to do it! Why regress all the way back to diapers? Shouldn't I offer some sort of bribe or reward? Chocolate? A complex sticker chart with a prize at the end?"

"Carolyn," he said, "there are a lot of things you can do for your children. You can send them to the best schools, you can make sure they take dance, soccer, and swimming lessons, you can even get them off a drunk driving charge! But, YOU CAN'T GO TO THE BATHROOM FOR THEM! Put her back in diapers, and when she is comfortable with school, she'll get back to her potty."

And she did. She got there, and her sister will too. So much about being a great pediatrician is being able to communicate and REALLY connect with parents. Dr. Heller had a VERY funny, informative and special way of communicating with me that ultimately made me a better parent. Because to care for children means to also care for their parents.

Parent Christine H. wrote,

I took Michael to see Dr. Heller because my son was not feeling well. During our visit, Dr. Heller received a call (Note: Dr. Heller always took phone calls immediately from parents.) from a mother whose child was not making bowel movements. The mother apparently did not know what to do and asked Dr. Heller about some bowel movement clinic at a hospital. Dr. Heller said he could send her child there but that the child would come out of that place with more of a problem than when the child went in. Dr. Heller then went on to explain that there are four areas of control with children 1.eating 2.sleeping 3.talking and 4.going to the bathroom. He then proceeded to tell the woman that this was a control issue and she needed to act accordingly. He told her not to worry if the child refused to go to the bathroom with this story "You have never heard of a terrorist going in a plane and saying 'I have not had a bowel movement in several days. If you don't do what I tell you I will blow up" have you?" This was another one of Dr. Heller's stories that brought the message home. He had to be extreme in his message to combat all the books and information that mothers are reading.

The Slippery Step of Peeing

Parent Yasmine K. wrote,

My favorite lesson from Dr. Danny was his explanation to my three year old daughter about how peeing properly would help her from getting a urinary tract infection. He brought out a copy of a wood cut by Rembrandt, showing a woman leaning against a tree while peeing. He explained to my daughter how people used to pee a long time ago, and how it was much better for your body. My daughter had been sitting on the toilet with her pants around her ankles, pressing her legs together and trapping the urine. He told her to sit on the toilet facing backwards—peeing like a boy. We went home and she was excited to try it. Not only did it feel better, she was very excited to see just where the pee was coming from! I forgot to tell her daycare providers about her change in toilet habits. I got a call about her refusal to face forward on the toilet. She emphatically told them that this is how Dr. Danny wanted her to pee, and this is how she was going to do it! She didn't have any more urinary problems as long as she followed his instructions.

About Teenagers and Drugs

Parent Doreen B. wrote,

At Justin's last physical (at age 16), Dr. Dan told Justin that if he ever thought of using drugs, to come to see Dr. Dan because Dr. Dan had a lot better ones and most teenagers who do drugs are depressed or have something else going on.

About Struggling with a Disability

Parent Doreen B. wrote,

When we learned Justin was dyslexic around age 14, Dr. Dan pointed out to Justin that his neurologist was also dyslexic and that Dr. Dan himself was. Dr. Dan related his the story of his own school life, and how he was going to be an auto mechanic because he was having such a hard time in school, and how his mother convinced him to stay in high school, and to try college and the rest is history … This was a great up-lifter for Justin and his parents to see how successful Justin could also be someday.

A Typical Wellness Visit with Dr. Heller

Robert and Patricia L. wrote,

"Do you always wear your bike helmet when you ride your bike?"

"Can you pick a booger out of your nose and flick it across the room?"

"Can you count from one to one hundred in three seconds? You can't? I can: 1 to 100! See!"

"Can you take a number and divide it?" [Dr. Heller then pulls out a piece of paper and writes a number on it; he rips the paper in half from top to bottom] "Long division!" [He rips the paper again from side to side] "Short division!"

"Have you ever slept **over** a friend's house? No? I don't blame you. It makes much more sense to sleep **inside** your friend's house."

"Do you drink lots of milk? Did you know that all that business about drinking milk is propaganda? You can get all the calcium you need from eating broccoli."

"Always wear socks when you travel. Why? I'll tell you why. I was on a trip to China. When I went into the airport bathroom, there wasn't any toilet paper. I couldn't call for help, because I don't speak Chinese, so I was pretty glad I was wearing socks because they are expendable, if you know what I mean."

Parent Linda Y. wrote,

We still laugh about the hats. What fun they were! The potty training hat was one of our favorites. And if there wasn't an appropriate hat—which didn't happen often—the guy had other props! When Mike turned 3 years old, Dan asked him how he celebrated his birthday and Mike told him about the pirate party. Dan grabbed his giant pencil as a telescope and jumped on top of his desk pulling Mike up with him, screaming, "Ahoy Matie! Can you see them coming down Route 9? Let's pillage and plunder." And the routine went on and on.

When Mike was about 5 years old, the question of the visit was what would you do if you came home and your mother was unconscious and on the floor. "Call 911," Mike said. "Yes!" proclaimed Dr. Heller, "You are much smarter than the last kid, who said he would sing, "Ding, dong, the witch is dead!"

We will always remember:
the crazy outfits
ankle weights
the sight of Dan driving by us on his bike with his beanie helmet
his good advice
the way he saved our friend's daughter when she had meningitis
his knowledge and caring
the way he could stop all antics when we were really worried about something.

Parent Lisa P. C. wrote,

In the course of a well visit, Dr. Dan asked my six-year-old, "Do you know all your letters? Can you throw a ball and catch a ball? Do you know the number to call in case of an emergency? Can you pick your nose and flick the booger across the room?"

I thought that the medical student would faint! Dr. Dan then explained that if a kid did not crack-up at this question as my kid had, that it showed Dr. Dan that something could be seriously wrong—either developmentally or emotionally.

Parent Rebekah S. wrote,

At last year's annual checkup, Dr. Heller interviewed the kids in his office, as usual. And, as usual, it was enjoyable for all of us. He asked my 5 year old daughter where her brain was, and she responded that it was in her head. Dr Heller then noted, "Good. It's moved up. Last year it was in your neck."

He asked my 9 year old son if he had ever slept over anyone's house, and Elias answered that he had. Dr. Heller's response was, "Oh, you shouldn't do that. It's very dangerous. You could roll off the roof." He then proceeded to tell us that every time he flies past Washington, D.C., he makes a point of falling asleep, so he can say that he's slept over the White House!

Parent Jamie L. wrote,

Each time we visited for our annual exams for my three boys, Dr. Heller had us in stitches! Dr. Heller's mellow and comical approach to caring for kids and their developmental milestones were similar to my own (except I'm not as funny). When my son, Daniel began puberty, the delicate issue of his pubic hair and penile "growth spurt" were turned into such a hoopla we were all beside ourselves. When he referred to Daniel's inevitable masturbation as a mass murder similar to the work of Hitler, Daniel was literally crying from laughter (and no doubt some embarrassment).

About Speaking Multiple Languages

Parent Katherine D. wrote,

Dr. Heller constantly advised me at EVERY visit with my 3 children to continue speaking Greek to them. "Their minds are like sponges", he would tell me. "English is around them everywhere but to learn a second language in life is invaluable."

He would ask them "Ti Kanis", which means How are you?

About Drinking Milk

Nancy's cousin Ben Darr said in his bar mitzvah speech,

I also want to mention my cousin Danny Heller who died this year shortly after his 60th birthday. While I may not have the guts to wear a cap with a propeller on it all the time, I admired his commitment to pediatrics, to family, to enjoying life and showing others a good time. He stuck to his principles even if he **was** the only doctor who believed kids don't need milk.

About ADD

Parent Joan W. wrote,

When our daughter was diagnosed with ADD, Dr. Dan didn't bore or overwhelm her with the usual psychobabble. He congratulated her on her survival skills, describing how early humans (and squirrels even today) needed to extend their attention in numerous directions in order to remain safe from environmental dangers.

Friend and school principal Carol S. wrote,

> The conversation I had with Dan about ADD kids is what I <u>always</u> share with parents. Dan said there is nothing wrong with ADD kids. They are wired for the world as it used to be—when being alert to distraction meant you were the person most likely to survive. School is an invention that runs counter to these kids. However, since school is where kids need to be, we need to help them adjust.
>
> Dan framed things in terms of what was inherently right about a child. Small wonder his patients and their parents loved him so much. Unconditional acceptance and respect are in short supply these days. Dan was the exception.

Dr. Dan's Notes about ADD

Question: How can I tell if my child has attention deficit disorder?

Answer: You can't, and neither can your health-care provider!

This question comes up frequently from parents, daycare providers, and teachers, regarding children they know from two years of age and right up to twenty and beyond: Who has attention deficit disorder or attention-deficit/hyperactivity disorder (ADD/ADHD)?

A pediatrician's response to a parent is usually (1) you cannot make the diagnosis until you are in second grade or (2) you need to go to a learning disability clinic for a complete evaluation. A complete evaluation means various psychometric and educational testing, which, unfortunately, is not covered by most insurance and which schools are hard pressed to provide.

Besides, after $1,800 to $2,400 worth of testing, the results never say, "Yes, your child has ADD." Rather, the answer is usually "He may have ADD" or "He may do better on stimulant medications." Currently, there is no test, no brain wave, no cranial ultrasound, no cranial scan, and no one can say definitively that a child has ADD.

Let's get back to basics. Humans have been on earth for seventy thousand years. For the first forty thousand years, we were hunter-gatherers and then became more agrarian. The human species were not only hunter-gatherers, but we were also hunted.

How does this relate to ADD? If you want to see the ultimate ADD/ADHD animal, think about a squirrel. A squirrel runs up the pole and then down, along the wire and then back, picks up an acorn then drops it, always moving and never seemingly focused. Why? The answer here is simple. The squirrel that focuses on only one thing quickly becomes dinner for birds from the sky, snakes on the ground, larger mammals, and, today, are victims of automobiles.

We humans were in the same boat. The cave person who could sit and "focus" on one thing easily became dinner for a saber-toothed tiger or a boa constrictor. Rather, we were imprinted with the ability to focus on many things at once.

We were made to notice odors in the air, noises in the brush, and movements in our peripheral vision so that we could survive. Knowing whether the noise behind you was that of a rabbit or that of a boa constrictor lays the difference between your *having* lunch or your *being* lunch. In fact, we are genetically mammals with multiple input abilities (MIA). We are capable of using our sight, hearing, smell, touch, and taste all the time and all at once in order to survive. Without having MIA, we would not be here today.

So when did MIA become ADD? When did this terrific ability to focus on multiple inputs become a problem? Today a child must sit in a classroom and needs, by modern standards, to deny all other inputs and *focus* on just one thing. In school, a child needs to block the peripheral vision, the sounds from outside, the unusual odors, and his sixth senses and simply *unifocus*.

It's important to keep in mind that school is an invention of our modern society, and it's important to realize that labeling a child as having a deficit or disorder may not be fair to the child when he has a problem in the school environment. The real problem for the educator, the parent, the child, and the provider is how we can help the child with MIA block the inputs that do not contribute to his modern-day education. We would have the same problem if we were trying to survive on a desert island trying to get the *focused* child to notice his surroundings and be a hunter. It basically is the environment that defines whether the ability to *unifocus* versus *multifocus* is a problem.

So how can we best determine which child needs help in accommodating to his environment? The best source is the teacher. Fortunately, most children are able to master their MIA for a sufficient amount of time to follow the curriculum and get educated. Teachers are usually the first to notice the child who has a problem blocking external inputs. About one quarter of the children who meet today's criteria for ADD have other underlying problems. Children with behavior disorders, psychiatric problems, and developmental delays overlap children who seem unable to focus. In fact, as noted earlier, the screening evaluations, while unable to define who has ADD, are able to identify children with these other types of problems.

The child who has no definitive diagnosis may be the one who will benefit by treatment with stimulant drugs. In fact, the only way to tell if a child's focus on school work will improve is to give a trial on this type of medication.

As noted from the start, neither you nor the health-care provider can tell if a given child has ADD/ADHD. The bottom line is to have a screening for a behavioral or psychiatric problem as a first step in evaluating a child whose teachers have identified as having a problem. The second step is to give a monitored trial on medication, realizing that we are not treating a disease or disorder but rather throwing a life preserver to a child in a hostile environment.

About Eating Disorders: Anorexia, Bulimia, and Obesity

When I was in medical school, only a few minutes of one lecture in psychiatry were spent on the topics of anorexia and bulimia. These were rare conditions that a young doctor was unlikely to encounter. The causes were poorly understood, and treatment was very difficult.

By the 1980s, eating disorders had become the topic of grand rounds; and many lectures were presented to update practicing physicians on the signs and symptoms of anorexia and bulimia. Making the diagnosis of an eating disorder is, in fact, fairly easy. Strict criteria exist as to the percentage below normal body weight that an individual must have to meet the criteria. Besides the direct measure of weight, the biochemical and metabolic derangements associated with eating disorders can give us a laboratory means of making the diagnosis. Certain findings on a physical exam and a mental status exam and electrocardiograms also assist in confirming the presence of an eating disorder. Yes, we have gotten very good at making the diagnosis.

Unfortunately, despite our excellence in making the diagnosis, our ability to prevent and treat these disorders has not improved much over the years. I have found very few psychiatrists, psychologists, or social workers who are able to turn these kids around. Our success rate at curing eating disorders is really rather poor.

All too often, I have seen an anorexic or bulimic child become a chronically obese child after therapy. Similarly, I have watched some very obese children become anorexic children with our treatment protocols.

One role of a pediatrician is to be a detective. Doctors take pride in their detective work. We enjoy the challenge. However, when I make the diagnosis of anorexia or bulimia, I am not proud. If a child has an eating disorder, I, in part, feel that I have to blame myself. Eating disorders do not develop overnight in the pre-adolescent or adolescent years. I am convinced that the seeds of this problem are not only societal but also relate to our pediatric advice about feeding and nutrition. I believe that we have helped to provide the groundwork that creates the road to eating disorders.

When I began practice, my colleague was of the old school on nutrition. Each patient was given a written note on what food to eat, when to eat it, and how much. "If you don't eat this or that, you won't get to have dessert or watch TV."

Subsequently, nutrition and dietician professions flourished with endless advice on how to get a child to eat "balanced" meals. Of course, those "balanced" meals seemed to change from year to year as some new theory came along. I watched as the food pie (a circle) changed into the food pyramid (a triangle). I watched the National Dairy Association plaster my children's kindergarten and grade-school classrooms with posters of milk and dairy products. At the same time, my cardiologist told me to cut out milk and dairy foods after my heart attack.

Ask yourself this question, why are eating disorders on the rise in a nation with so much food and so much food advice? I have come to the realization that the advice must not work!

Ask yourself why a cow never drinks milk, only water, and eats only vegetables and yet is healthy. Ask yourself why an elephant (which is much larger than you and me combined) eats grass and tree bark and yet is not osteoporotic or calcium deficient. Ask yourself why a lion or tiger eats only meat (no vegetables) and drinks just water and yet is faster and stronger than you or me. Ask yourself why human beings were, for forty thousand years, hunter-gatherers, eating fish, meat, roots, and berries and drinking water and survived quite well.

If you ask enough of these questions, you begin to realize that mammals do quite fine on this planet as vegetarians with water as a liquid and no rules. Do you really think the caveman went through stage one, stage two, stage three and stage four foods for the introduction of food to his newborn? More likely, cave people ate whatever they could find; and then they chewed some up and spit it out and offered it to their babies. As that cave baby grew up, he, too, ate whatever was available.

So why has there been an increase in the incidence of eating disorders in America today? Do you really think that cave children ate food and then ran behind a tree to throw up? Or that cave children refused to eat after a hunt? Do you think that anorexia and bulimia are major problems in Ethiopia or Somalia today where there is famine and starvation?

"If it ain't broke, don't fix it" is an oft-used phrase. "If it is broke, fix it" must be a reasonable corollary. I think our advice over the past forty years to parents has not had the intended result. We create a pressure on parents that they are only "good" if they ensure "good" nutrition. Our advice has encouraged parents to become embattled with their infants and toddlers over feeding issues; the fallout comes years later as severe eating issues.

It is time that we take a giant step backward. Let's not make such a big issue over what is "good" and what is "bad" when it comes to food. We should offer our infants and toddlers a variety and not be concerned if they don't want everything. This is not to say that parents offer junk food. Infants do not know what is junk food. There is no law that says you have to have junk food in the house. There is no law that says dessert must come after every meal.

Remember that, in a food fight, your infant or toddler will win. If parents do not get embattled from the start, I am convinced that there will be no battles later. *The answer to eating disorders is in their prevention and not in their treatment.* The treatments, as noted above, are not very successful. We would be far better off to practice preventive measures; the best measure is to relax the rules about feeding and nutrition.

If your infant or toddler is growing well at his regular checkups, then how he achieved that growth does not matter. Spending time discussing how much or how little he ate does not matter. If he ate nothing and grew normally, what can I say but congratulations—you saved a lot on food money. And if he ate everything in the house and is not overweight, I can only say that's great.

About Death

Cheryl W., niece of Nancy's sister, Susan, wrote,

After Susan died, I remember being at your home after the memorial service. I was young and in college then and struggling terribly with my Aunt Susan's death. I ended up sitting on the floor way upstairs in some corner of your house. I was hysterically crying and I was trying to get away from all of the people downstairs who were smiling, laughing and seemingly to me, having a party.

Well, there I was, pathetic, alone and hysterical. All of a sudden, Danny came and sat next to me. He could see how upset I was and the two of us started talking. I was struggling so much with all of the "happy noise" at Susan's memorial gathering and I told him so. He said very kindly that basically death was a part of life. He explained to me that everyone was sad, hurt, upset and distraught over Susan's death, but that we were here and living and we, as hard as it is, needed to celebrate Susan's life, how she lived and the people she touched. Then he put back on his hat, smiled and together we came back downstairs to celebrate Susan's life because he was right and Susan would have wanted us to be smiling and laughing.

Well, sadly, here we are again—mourning over a loved one. But as I cry, I think of Danny the man, the father, the friend, the joker, the doctor, and I think how lucky I am to have had such a person touch my life. I also remember well his lesson and I know he would want us all to try and not be sad but to celebrate Dr. Daniel Heller's life and how he lived. He touched, cared for and helped so many people—what a truly amazing man.

Index

978-0-595-67964-5
0-595-67964-1

Printed in the United States
70708LV00004B/115-399